The Power
of Hope

A Doctor's Perspective

Prepared under

the auspices of the

Program for Humanities

in Medicine, Yale University

School of Medicine

Yale University Press

New Haven & London

Portions of this book previously appeared in Doctors, Patients, and Placebos (Yale University Press, 1986).

The poem "When You Come into My Room," by Stephen A. Schmidt (JAMA 276:512, 1996), copyright 1996, American Medical Association, is excerpted with permission of the publisher.

The information and suggestions contained in this book are not intended to replace the advice or services of your physician or other caregiver. Rather, they are editorial comments from my doubtless idiosyncratic perspective of fifty years in medicine. Because each person and each medical situation is unique, consult your own physician for answers to your questions or for evaluations of any symptoms you have and certainly before you take any medications, mainstream or alternative.

I have attempted to make this book as accurate and up-to-date as possible, but it may nevertheless contain errors, omissions, or material that is out-of-date at the time you read it. Neither the author nor the publisher has any legal responsibility or liability for errors, omissions, out-of-date material, or the reader's application of any medical information or advice contained in this book.

Designed by Sonia L. Scanlon.
Set in Joanna type by
dix!, Syracuse, New York.
Printed in the United States of America.

CIP data are at the back of the book.

A catalogue record for this book is available from the British Library.

The paper in this book meets the guidelines for permanence and durability of the Committee on Production Guidelines for Book Longevity of the Council on Library Resources.

10   9   8   7   6   5   4   3   2   1

To the patients who,
in sickness and in health,
have taught me so much.

Contents

Preface

In 1955, when I came to Connecticut to set up the first gastrointestinal unit at Yale University medical school, there were only five gastroenterologists in the state, which then had slightly fewer than three million people. In those days, I saw patients with common diseases, like cancer of the colon or stomach, colitis, and pancreatitis, and with other problems that called for a specific diagnostic approach and standard therapy. In the four decades since then, the population of Connecticut has grown only slightly, to something over three million, but the number of gastroenterologists has soared, to more than two hundred. The ubiquity of gastroenterologists has changed the kinds of patients who come to a university physician. Many people whom I now see complain of pain for which their doctors cannot easily find an origin despite the myriad imaging studies inflicted upon them.

Pain, sometimes in the form of tribulation, has become a central concern in my consultative practice. I have learned, partly from the flowering of controlled clinical trials, how readily some pains disappear, as quickly after a placebo as after an active drug, but I have also learned how many pains persist unexplained, wrapping their victims in persistent anguish and sometimes torment.

During a sabbatical in California in the 1980s, I had the leisure to wonder about the relief of pain by placebos and about what that suggested about clinical practice, patient-physician relationships, and other therapeutic and diagnostic concerns. The result was a book, *Doctors, Patients, and Placebos,* published by Yale University Press in 1986. When Dr. Joseph Jacobs, then head of the Alternative Medicine Office at the National Institutes of Health in Washington, D.C., suggested that the book deserved wider distribution in paperback form, I was happy to update matters, rethink the subject, and open up the discussion. The result is the book you now hold in your hands.

In this new book I emphasize the close relation between self-help, caring, placebos, and the healing power of nature. For the relief of pain and suffering and for the energizing of self-help and self-reliance, patients can help themselves, and healers with confidence in their patients, who care for their patients, can help even more. But there are no longer any miracles. Throughout this book I emphasize the distinctions between *disease,* what the doctor can find and see, and *illness,* what the patient feels. It is important to remember the difference as we talk about what doctors and treatments can do.

In *Doctors, Patients, and Placebos* are listed the persons to whom I was indebted for help and ideas, and my ideas today still owe much to them. Here I offer special thanks to Priscilla Norton, who read the new manuscript from beginning to end and offered many valuable suggestions. Stefan Weiss, as a third- and fourth-year Yale College student, worked with me on philosophical and technical aspects of placebos; I thank him for his energetic help and discussions, and I wish him well in medical school. Patricia Perona, administrative assistant to the Program for Humanities in Medicine at Yale, has had many wise suggestions for which I have taken the credit in this book. Nikola M. Biller, who has just received her medical degree from the University of Erlangen, reviewed the entire manuscript while she was a visiting scholar at Yale as a fellow of the Studienstiftung German Academic Exchange Council. She, too, tested my ideas and made many useful suggestions. The Center for Advanced Studies in Behavioral Studies at Stanford University gave me a sabbatical refuge some years ago that still energizes me. I am especially grateful to Yale University School of Medicine and its various deans and chairs who have left me to follow my own inclinations over the past four decades. I also thank Jean Thomson Black of Yale University Press for her editorial skills and Mary

Pasti, also of the press, for her queries, redactions, and doubts about elusive portions of my text. Of course I thank Marian Spiro, my partner of forty-seven years, who pruned my pomposity and puts up with my spiritual arrogance. And I thank Joe Jacobs, now happily in Vermont, who set this enterprise in motion.

Because I intend this book as much for general readers as for physicians and medical students, I have pruned the academic paraphernalia vigorously. There are two reference lists. The first, alphabetical one gives references cited by author or name in the text. The second, not alphabetical, gives additional sources for studies mentioned and occasionally for quotations not otherwise attributed that have contributed to the ideas in this book. These sources are listed in the order in which they are pertinent.

More and more people manage their own care by checking out the Internet's prodigious health and medical resources. They can find sites labeled epilepsy, lupus, Parkinson's; others called American Medical Association Home Page or The Virtual Hospital; and doctors billing themselves as "H. Spiro, gastroenterologist." Curbed of the chance to talk to their doctor, who needs "heavy patient traffic" to keep income up, even people with obscure diseases explore chat lines, e-mail, home pages, and all the other paraphernalia of electronic information. I hope this book will provide a more leisurely and comprehensive—shall I say "holistic?"—view of medicine and medical practices.

The Power of Hope

To relieve pain, more than once I have prescribed placebos in what I hope was an honest way. To help patients with symptoms that I do not immediately recognize, and fear I will never be able to categorize—such as weakness and lassitude that do not come from depression—I have suggested regular injections of one thousand micrograms of vitamin B_{12}. I tell such patients, "I'm going to advise some B_{12} injections. They have helped many other patients, but I cannot explain why they work and I cannot promise that they will work. Many people tell me they feel better and stronger afterward, and I hope you will, too." Such prescriptions have helped many people and, I hope, harmed no one.

I believe that such shots lessen anxiety and give hope and new strength because my words give patients hope that the shots will help them. In trying to help this way, I do not feel that I have deceived anyone. Imagine my surprise to have an ethicist suggest that in using *any* placebo I was deceiving patients—a rebuke that started my review of placebos and how they work.

Placebos are important for what they do and for what they say about the patient-physician relationship. Now that alternative or complementary medicine is so widespread, placebos also stand in for those new-old approaches to healing: they hint at self-healing and the mind-body puzzle.[1] Alternative medical practices can help our overmedicalized society by lightening the burden on patients undergoing endless medical tests. Like placebos, they tell us of the magic and mystery of life, reminding us that there are some answers that science cannot provide.

Placebos depend on patients for their action more than on doctors, because their primary effect is psychological, in the renewed energy that faith, hope, and expectation may bring. That in turn may or may not bring bodily improvement—how we do not know. Still, at a time when medical practice has turned so technical in aim, placebos highlight what self-help and self-healing, so important to alternative medicine, can do for those who are sick. That is what this book is all about: helping sick people.

Science and Medicine: Cure over Care

Thinking about placebos has made me reexamine the emphasis on science that characterizes modern medicine: physicians learn how to cure but little about how to care. They learn to detect and treat diseases, especially the acute ones they see in the hospital. Care is often ignored. One vowel makes such a big difference: cure is directed at disease, and care at patients. The effects of placebos make doctors and nurses think about their patients as much as their patients' organs.

The scientific approach to human disease—the biomedical or molecular model that has brought so many cures—cannot answer all patients' needs. Disease is what the doctor finds; but that is quite different from illness, what the patient feels. Placebos help illness; they relieve suffering. Whether they can affect the pathophysiological events that underlie disease is not clear.

Looking Versus Listening

Placebos assert the power of community, the ability of one person to help another. That claim may seem self-serving, but now, under managed care programs, all physicians are regarded as identical units to be controlled by rule books. It is important to remember that people are comforted by people. I place the benefit of placebos squarely with patients and find in everyday people the strength of modern self-help movements. Placebos celebrate caring and healing and remind all of us, doctors and patients, that we are not alone. Not all anecdotes are equal, but there are good lessons for the mainstream in alternative medical practices and in the "black box" of placebos.

Good physicians listen to the stories that their patients tell, and then interpret the findings of X-rays and other images in the context of those complaints. They remember that relief is something doctors can always provide, even when they are not sure what is wrong.

The metaphors by which we live define and limit what we do, and they are crucial for physicians. Many modern physicians see themselves only as scientists and never as poets. One reason why doctors overtreat and overstudy and do not always talk with, or listen to, their patients is that they are too busy looking at organs and laboratory findings. The eye rules the ear in current medical practice.

Modern doctors want hard data and hard copy, visual evidence or at least some numbers. Physicians have adopted a precise attitude toward tobacco and alcohol, recording the pack-years of tobacco smoked and grams of alcohol consumed, but they pay little attention to personal, cultural, and social aspects of life, which are hard to measure.

Existential Pain

Because I do no procedures, I see many patients with what I call existential pain and others call somatization. Typical is a thirty-four-year-old Hispanic woman who showed up at the Primary Care Clinic at Yale. Her doctors wanted me to rule out H. pylori, a bacterial infection of the stomach, as the cause of her abdominal pain; she had also been to the gynecologist for chronic pain in her pelvis and to a scattering of other specialists. She spoke no English, so through an interpreter I learned that her alcoholic husband had no job and that he beat her. Three pregnancies had eventuated in miscarriages; the fourth left her with a daughter in a wheelchair who required much attention for bladder and bowel problems. I wondered how much the primary care physicians expected bacteria to contribute to her troubles.

Patients and Doctors

During my medical career, medicine has exchanged a professional for a business model, and other new issues have surfaced; among them are cost restraints, the overuse of technology, and new ethical questions sprung from new medical skills. Examining my use of placebos has entailed some reflections on how physicians and patients treat each other in this new environment and has led me to consider how alternative medical practices bring their benefits. Modern medical culture often mistakes the means—science—for the ends: caring for patients. Technology is overused because doctors expect to find an answer to every problem if they only look hard enough with the right instruments. Physicians learn to find the cause of a symptom before treating it, because relieving a symptom like pain without ascertaining its cause is derided as bad medicine. Handing out pills without thinking about the reasons for the complaints will lead to trouble, but sometimes, when doctors know their patients, providing relief, instead of identifying causes, may be enough. That was easy long ago, but it is much harder in our mobile society, where strangers must care for strangers.

Psychosomatic Medicine

A gastroenterologist educated at Harvard in the 1940s, I gave up endoscopy—looking into the stomach or bowel with tubes—in the 1960s because I was sure that trained technicians could do that as easily and more cheaply. Consequently, I see many people with complaints that have not yielded to the more intrusive and narrowly focused diagnostic endeavors of my endoscopic colleagues. I have had much occasion to think about patients and pain, doctors and placebos, and the site of that existential pain mentioned earlier.

The psychosomatic theories of those times were best expressed in the book *Psychosomatic Medicine*. "The physician who prescribes placebos, in whatever form, is not consciously dishonest. He wants to help his patient. He knows his patient expects drug treatment. He is aware of the resistance of the patient to the idea that his symptoms are the result of emotional conflict. He (the doctor) has seen the beneficial effects of suggestion by placebos in other cases and hopes that the same thing will happen again. When he runs out of placebos the patient runs out on him" (Weiss and English). Norman Cousins, whose account of his illness will be reviewed in Chapter 8, many years later commented, "I have wondered, in fact, about the relative absence of attention given the placebo in contemporary medicine. . . . I was absolutely convinced, at the time I was deep in my illness, that intravenous doses of ascorbic acid could be beneficial—and they were. It is quite possible that this treatment—like everything else I did—was a demonstration of the placebo effect. If so, it would be just as important to probe into the nature of this psychosomatic phenomenon as to find out if ascorbic acid is useful in combatting a high sedimentation rate" (Cousins 1976). One of my colleagues, the psychiatrist Jay Katz, has similarly observed that "if placebos were to be acknowledged as effective in their own right, it would expose large gaps in medicine's and doctors' knowledge about underlying mechanisms of care and relief from suffering" (Katz).

The Three Stages of Modern Medicine

There was a time when that synthesis of social, psychic, and physical influences collectively known as psychosomatic medicine promised to teach doctors a mainstream view of patients that was holistic as well as scientific. Psychosomatic medicine grew out of a larger movement that flourished earlier in the century, social medicine. At Yale in the 1920s, the Institute of Human Relations, founded and fostered by Milton Winternitz, dean of Yale University School of Medicine, and James Rowland Angell, president of the university, tried to insert the social sciences and psychology into the medical curriculum to encourage physicians to consider more than the bodies of their patients. The building that they created outlasted them but now houses a laboratory for genetics. All that remains of the dreams of the 1920s is the old name carved over the main entrance to the medical school.

The failure of that vision of social medicine underlines the faultiness of the model that modern physicians have followed and the value of the postmodern ideal of what physicians should do. Physicians once saw themselves as *practitioners* at the bedside and later as *clinicians* in a hospital; now, for the most part, they learn to act like *scientists*, or at least like *technicians*, in a laboratory. Practitioners see the patient as a person, in whom all parts should be working in harmony. Clinicians concentrate on diseases and biological lesions, regarding the very sick in intensive care units as cases. Carried over into a doctor's office or clinic, this attitude can lead to misunderstanding between patients and physicians, especially when the doctor is too busy to be the listening healer that we all want.

Scientific or laboratory medicine—which has dominated medical training for the past half century—turns the physician into a scientist, someone who traces the twists and turns of amino acids rather than considering the whole patient. Diseases begin in cells, an approach that Rudolf Virchow, the great nineteenth-century pathologist, called cellular pathology; genetic engineering illustrates how close medical science today is to the cellular therapy that he foresaw. Take as an example the treatment of peptic ulcer, vastly easier than before, now that over-the-counter agents block the output of acid from the stomach; even more sophisticated ones inhibit the "proton pump" within the cell, and antibiotics bid fair to abolish the ulcer's return. Reducing stress and modifying the diet to cure and prevent ulcers is much harder than swallowing pills and potions—no wonder medical practice focuses on biologically detectable organic lesions and their biochemical and immunological deviations, for they are easier to remedy than the social, cultural, and economic issues that cause so many medical problems. This "reductionism" still rules medical practice.

Modern doctors emphasize finding the perturbations of disease, especially in its subcellular disturbances. Scientist-physicians look, but rarely listen. Patients, however, have not changed; they want to get better, and most would like to talk more to their doctors. Most of us patients like to think that we are unique, more than just a collection of data or another case.

Of course, there is more to life than medicine, and it may be arrogant for physicians to assume that someone who comes for treatment of a specific complaint wants anything more. I want my barber to trim my hair, but not to shave my beard because he thinks I will appear younger. Physicians have to be careful about taking on responsibility that they have not been asked to assume.

Modern and Postmodern Medicine

Modern medicine began with the success of Pasteur's vaccine against rabies and the development of an antitoxin for diphtheria; the continuing victories in the war against bacteria provide the reason why military metaphors dominate medical images. Once salvarsan came along for syphilis, doctors hoped for magic bullets to cure cancer, heart disease, and even the common cold. The current war against H. pylori as the cause of stomach ulcers offers a new example: if antibiotics can cure an ulcer, there is no need to discuss the stresses that may have brought it on.

Modern medicine, or biomedicine, has been so successful in the management of many acute disorders that doctors have a hard time admitting that they are less good at helping patients with chronic problems that may require a more holistic approach. Rheumatism, allergies, back and belly pain, and high blood pressure fall somewhere between disease and illness, and all are problems that alternative medical practitioners help very well, unlike cancer and depression.

The Flexner Report in the early twentieth century, discussed in Chapter 11, put biomedicine in control and channeled medical practice into mainstream rivers, damming up alternative contributions (including abolishing most schools where women were learning medicine). The growth of specialization over the past forty years has made it hard for mainstream doctors to treat patients with complaints that are not reflected in images from their X-ray, CAT scan, or other machines. That is one reason why alternative medicine has become primary care medicine at its very best, addressing the problems for which scientific medicine cannot provide solutions.

Postmodernism represents a revolution against the dominant theme and conviction of the twentieth century: that Western civilization should provide the goals for the whole world. In the 1960s we saw the rise of women's rights, the black struggle for equal rights, and a loss of faith in many institutions. Postmodernism, as it has come to be called, had its beginning in literary deconstructionism, which called for thinking less about what is said and more about what has not been said, looking at the margins of the text as well as the words themselves. One consequence of that revolt has been multiculturalism and diversity, which represent a major fount of alternative medicine.

Postmodern medicine must be seen in that broader social context. It looks new, but it is a return to very old ideas, some in the United States going back to the egalitarian era of Andrew Jackson. The pendulum, having swung from reason to intuition, will doubtless swing back again. Not yet widely recognized as part of the postmodern movement, alternative medicine has been growing slowly without a uniform set of principles, partly because health rather than disease is its subject. Health is so hard to define that difficulties arise when doctors aim at health rather than disease.

Health and Disease

In postmodern accounts of healing, disease and illness have become equal. "I feel better" has become equivalent to "I am cured," but the two are very different, and that is at the base of many conflicts between modern and postmodern physicians. For modern practitioners of scientific medicine *cure* and *care* remain distinct, and *healing* is a term used largely outside mainstream circles. *Healing* remains mystical when used to mean "helping body, mind, and spirit." I do not demean this usage, but to heal is not to cure, as modern doctors use the word.

The conflict between practitioners of alternative medicine and more mainstream medicine comes from this difference between treating disease and illness. Modern medicine deals very well with acute problems like pneumonia and broken legs, but it is very much less helpful for the pain and depression caused by arthritis or the dyspepsia that grows with stress. Medical practice and health practice lie at opposite poles; medical school teaches about disease to students whose patients will want health.

As I breach the firewall between the mainstream medicine that I was raised in and the complementary alternative practices that were once forbidden, I grow more certain that it is not the specific process or technique that makes patients better but the time that the doctor spends with the patient. Technique versus time has also proved a major question for psychotherapy in the era of managed care. In that sense, placebos are not another form of alternative medicine but a surrogate for these other approaches, all of which have some final common pathway for their benefits. I believe there is nothing specific about these complementary approaches and that many enthusiasts mistake the technique that brings relief to be specific. Psychiatrists abandoning psychoanalysis wonder whether their training and skills are as important as they once thought or whether it is the hour—or half hour! —with the patient that does the trick. There are equally serious questions about the theories behind some complementary practices. Still, I sometimes dream that the psychosomatic medicine of my youth can become the behavioral medicine of the next millennium. Doctors will have to be more than a little eclectic, recognizing that a massage might be as helpful as a review of the past.

Placebos have led me to folk medicine, faith healing, and other arts still slightly disreputable in medical circles. Indeed, Andrew Weil has somewhere called placebos the secret shame of medicine. Placebos, like alternative medicine, remind doctors of the uncertain borders of medical work; anthropological reports of healing in other cultures attest to the many ways that different cultures explain disease or define what it means to be sick, explanations and definitions that can broaden Western ideas of what doctors do.

Science, the Foundation of Medicine

Science remains the basis of modern medical practice, and I will stand on firm scientific ground as I examine placebos and their effects, as well as the claims of alternative practices. Medical practice is stretched by the tensions between science and intuition; the lens of the placebo has helped me focus on some of those strains.

Predictability and Reproducibility

Let me emphasize the importance of a rational, skeptical approach to claims for placebos and alternative healing. It is easy to rip single observations from their context, to use them as stepping stones to unwarranted conclusions. In writing about the claim for acupuncture, for example, the late Peter Skrabanek, a Hungarian living in Ireland, put it well: "What is at issue is the complex problem of demarcation between science and quackery, between honest search for truth and unscrupulous exploitation of human suffering."

Anything can be made to sound logical. It is easy to become so entranced with miracles or magic that one casts aside weighty, cumbersome scientific principles. But scientific principles must apply to evaluating the unknown, even placebos and the plausible.

Observation and Explanation

Medicine has come to look with disdain on the purely anecdotal. Still, if something happens once, it can happen again. Knowledge comes from classifying and testing hypotheses. Physicians need to ask how placebos help people and when, instead of regarding the unexplained improvements in health as a nuisance.

Until recently most physicians did not know how aspirin relieved pain even though they prescribed it and took it themselves. If they knew in the 1960s that aspirin raised the pain perception threshold, in the 1970s that it inhibited "prostaglandin synthetase," and in the 1980s that it originated from cell membranes, they understood its actions more and more specifically, but their practice remained unchanged. Even postmodern physicians recommend aspirin for far more than pain relief. Physicians try to ground their practice in scientific medicine. If it turns out that placebos relieve pain in part by stimulating endogenous endorphins or by activating rehearsed neutral networks, we still must ask whether knowing why placebos work justifies their use any more than simply knowing that they work.

Observation is not explanation. Classifying anecdotes of placebo miracles is not the same as explaining their mechanisms. But just because doctors do not yet know how placebos work, they need not avoid prescribing them. If physicians had awaited an explanation of how penicillin cured pneumonia instead of relying on clinical experience, they would have waited many years. Doctors could take X-rays to see some pneumonias vanish overnight, but penicillin was useless against viral pneumonia. Placebos do not work in all patients, so they could have concluded that penicillin was a placebo, resisted prescribing it, and let patients suffer or die. Analyzing when placebos are effective is as crucial as classifying pneumonias. Finding a biological explanation of how placebos work is desirable, but knowing that relief springs from faith will not make the question of deception redundant nor make lying to patients respectable.

Anything that directs the attention of patients away from their pain may help. Before my daughter Carolyn became a psychiatrist, she suggested that I could do without novocaine at the dentist's if I redirected my attention from my mouth. The technique worked, and, besides, I knew the pain would not last long. That redirection of attention and sometimes of imagination is abetted by many of the therapies that I will discuss in this book.

Forbidden Questions

There should be no forbidden questions. Because something cannot be explained by the reigning scientific paradigm is no reason to ignore it, but neither is that a reason to believe it. Heart and gene transplants and the revelations of neurobiology tempt us to direct our energies only toward the scientific frontier. Yet shadows can enlarge and cast into relief; at the margins of the known and the unknown, the measurable and the unmeasurable, the rational and the intuitive, much can be seen and learned. Placebos remind us that a good deal of what physicians do is not grounded in reason and may never need to be. The placebo makes us concentrate on the role of the physician and the patient in the healing process.

Who Should Read This Book

Contemplation of placebos and alternative medical practices and how they work has illuminated the goals of mainstream medical practice and education for me. Students study science to get into medical school; then they look for a good residency, or hospital internship, to learn how to manage seriously ill patients; and until very recently many residents aimed at a subspecialty with enough high-tech tools to give them the confidence of being effective in treating patients. After a decade or more of hospital training in disease diagnosis and treatment, physicians come out into the world of the sick and the worried well, where half the complaints that they hear prove to have no medical cause. They find themselves poorly prepared to deal with illness and pain except by turning complaints into diseases through their technological pursuits. Consideration of placebos as a nontechnological link between doctors and patients has made me encourage young people thinking about medical school to study art and anthropology as well as organic chemistry and physics.

This book is intended, then, to give lay readers a glimpse of the uncertainties in medicine, both mainstream and complementary. Medical interest groups have been responsible for much progress, but they have too zealously educated the public to expect quick cures for most diseases or to believe that enough money and resources will provide a cure for the disease of death. That is why patients demand too many tests for too many minor complaints. Perhaps reading this book will help the lay public to tolerate medical uncertainty, even for themselves.

The *placebo drama* has four parts: a physician gives what he or she believes to be an *inert material* to a *sick person*, and the *placebo effect* follows—symptoms improve. Hidden behind the curtains, the *placebo response*, which accounts for the improvements, gets little applause. I believe the placebo response to be caused mainly by a change in the patient's perception. The physician, the placebo, and the patient together bring about the relief of symptoms that we call the placebo effect. Oral medicines—pills or potions—are the usual placebos, but operations, injections, and even diagnostic and therapeutic maneuvers also may be placebos. Many patients feel better after taking a placebo, but that does not mean that their disease, if they have one, has improved, for relief of symptoms is *not* the same as cure of disease.[1]

The *Oxford English Dictionary* says that *placebo* was the name given to Vespers in the Office for the Dead because the first antiphonal response began with the Latin *placebo* ("I shall please"). Verse 9 of Psalm 116 in the King James version of the Bible goes, "I will walk before the Lord in the land of the living," but somehow an error turned "I will walk" into "I will please." So *placebo* gradually became a synonym for an inert or harmless medicine given to please the patient. In 1811 the term first came into use as "medicine prescribed more to please the patient than for its therapeutic effectiveness."

Henry Beecher, a Harvard professor who provided the foundation for most subsequent observations of the placebo and its effects, wrote of its common purpose "as a psychological instrument in the therapy of certain ailments arising out of mental illness, as a resource of the harassed doctor in dealing with a neurotic patient to determine the true effect of drugs apart from suggestion, in experimental work, as a device for eliminating bias not only on the part of the patients but also, when used as an unknown, of the observer, and, finally, as a tool of importance in the study of mechanisms of drug action" (Beecher 1955).[2] Placebos are used today in two ways: in clinical trials as a substitute for treatment and in practice as therapy. These are quite separate purposes.

Clinical Trials

To evaluate the effect of any proposed new treatment, controlled clinical trials are needed. To be controlled, a clinical trial must have four features: (1) random assignment of subjects to therapeutic or control groups, (2) a double-blind structure, (3) placebo control to minimize bias, and (4) enough subjects to satisfy statistical requirements specified beforehand. Let me give an example.

Duodenal Ulcer Trials

To find out whether a new drug relieves pain or speeds healing of duodenal ulcers, a group of patients each of whom has dyspepsia and an ulcer crater seen at endoscopy receive a new drug. Because duodenal ulcers tend to heal on their own with almost any treatment or even no treatment, patients taking a new drug must be compared to others who receive no treatment. If patients know what they are ingesting, any improvement might be psychological, thanks to their faith in a new wonder drug or the extra attention lavished on them by the doctors. A control group therefore receives an inactive substitute identical in appearance to the active drug. The substitute is called a placebo.

To be fair to all, patients are randomly chosen by computer to receive either drug or placebo. They are informed about the selection process beforehand. Because the enthusiasm of the physician heightens the benefit of a drug as part of the placebo effect, and because chagrin at receiving no therapy or the same old standby might worsen indigestion in the control patients, such trials are carried out "double-blind";

physicians and patients alike are ignorant of who receives which treatment.

Placebos in such trials also act as a measure of the natural tendency of an ulcer to heal, especially since just being cared for may speed natural healing. That is an important consideration in placebo healing.

Controlled trials brought their own surprises twenty years ago: almost 60 percent of ulcers healed in placebo takers and only a few more, about 70 percent, in the specific-drug takers. An observer who concluded that the drug, cimetidine, was as effective as it proved to be, might have wondered about that 60 percent. What was healing by placebo telling physicians about the medical arts and the need for medications? Could the benefit of the new drug be almost incidental to the symbolic nature of the interaction between physician and patient, however constrained by double-blind conventions?

In the excitement about the new drug, however, most investigators ignored the benefit of the placebo, even though patients who got the placebo did almost as well as those who were given the active agent. At two weeks ulcers were documented to have healed in 56 percent of patients receiving the active drug, significantly more than the 37 percent of patients receiving the placebo, but at other periods up to six weeks cimetidine and placebo proved equally effective. Although a number of theories explained away these observations, there was little discussion about the effect of the controlled trials themselves or the specific helpfulness of placebos.

The dramatic placebo response of patients with many other disorders—the anginal chest pain of heart disease among them—makes it hard to sort out how much relief comes from the dedicated attention that patients enrolled in such studies receive (and could likewise receive outside a study from an ordinary office visit), their hope that they are receiving the active drug, and the ceremony of participating in a study.

Observers have wondered whether patients in such studies who fear getting a placebo would be skeptical about the promised benefit from even the active drugs. After all, they point out, an analgesic gave more relief in a controlled trial when the patients knew that it was being compared with another active drug than when they knew it was being tested against a placebo. That suggests that expectation brings relief, a crucial contribution to the placebo effect. Telling patients who are given a placebo that they are receiving an active drug might help them, too, but that would be unethical.

That tells us that controlled clinical trials with placebos are really conditioning experiments: those who receive the active drug get relief and therefore reinforcement every time they take it because of its genuine therapeutic effects. In contrast, those who take the placebo get no such reinforcement, because the treatment they receive is without intrinsic effect. Comparing one active drug to another also gives reinforcement, which may be why such trials usually generate enthusiastic comparisons of a new drug with the tried and true.

Some hold that just being selected for a trial helps. To evaluate that possibility, Irving Kirsch suggests that a group of patients be given neither the treatment nor the placebo, so that their improvement or lack thereof will tell whether expectation contributes to the placebo effect. After all, college students who expect to get high on beer quite often do so on just one glass if everyone else around them is drinking. Another way of evaluating the effect of expectancy is to give all three groups a standard established treatment but different expectations of just how much better they will feel.

Spontaneous Remission

Spontaneous remissions must account for some of the celebrated triumphs of placebos and other medical practices, complementary and mainstream alike. Editors of journals and newspapers, as well as patients and doctors, prefer accounts of miracles to those of failures, which explains many ephemeral "breakthroughs" in the treatment of cancer that fill the news media year after year.

Hawthorne Effect

How an observer affects a study has been called the Hawthorne effect: increased attention brings its own benefit to those being watched. Factory workers were more efficient when they thought they were being observed, just as doctors in an emergency room who were told that they were being monitored did better than when they were observed secretly. Thinking that they were being observed made doctors and factory workers alike work harder and better, just as visiting a doctor helps patients relax and begin to improve.

Ethics of Placebos in Trials

The ethics of controlled trials with placebos has had so much discussion that no general rule is ever likely to be set. Everyone agrees that humans should never be treated as a means to an end, but in medical practice, decisions are made on a case-by-case basis, in a casuistry sometimes decried.

It is hard to justify giving a child a placebo instead of a proven vaccine, but it may not be unethical to use a placebo on an adult who runs a very, very small risk without treatment. Informed consent is the rule; the patient-subject must give the final assent.

Open trials of new medications—that is, trials in which physicians and patients know who gets the placebo and who the active drug—are still debated despite the preceding considerations. Physicians rightly point out that they want to find whether a new drug has any potential value before they enlist patients for a more rigorous study. But if an open trial gives the impression that the drug is very effective, continuing a placebo control can be criticized.

Very few have found fault with placebos in clinical trials, unless there are already drugs so effective that not taking them will harm patients. Placebo trials may benefit others more than they benefit the 50 percent of patients in the study who turn out to be controls. Investigators want, and the Food and Drug Administration (FDA) demands, firm statistical data; a comparison with a placebo will give a dramatic contrast between the effect of a new drug and the natural course of a disease. To compare a new drug with a proven one requires far more patients. To some extent, this is a social question: How many resources should be used to prove the marginal superiority of a new drug over an old one? Indeed, when the omission of treatment will not harm patients, one may ask whether the disease needs any treatment at all.

What about those volunteers who have only a fifty-fifty chance of receiving effective therapy? That depends on the disease under study. For lymphoma, for example, where modern therapy has proven so lifesaving, any proposed treatment must be compared to current methods. For uncomplicated duodenal ulcers, which are generally benign, placebo therapy in a trial seems ethical to me, but not many other doctors agree these days. Doubts linger about whether placebo trials are ethical when known therapy has minimal side effects and those of the new agent are unknown.

Importance of Placebo Controls

Comparing one drug with another already in use may lead researchers to accept drugs as effective when they are not very active at all. Ulcers heal spontaneously, as we have seen—20 percent did in a London study, 70 percent in a Swiss study, and from 50 to 60 percent in a U.S. study. Such studies remain pertinent even if the reasons for the healing remain unclear—whether something in the patients, in their doctors, or in the general expectation of a cure. In one very old study, antacids relieved ulcer pain 79 percent of the time in one hospital and only 17 percent of the time in another. In France, the placebo-healing rates were different for different physicians but were fairly constant over time.

All those reports tell us that people react differently to placebos, whether from expectation or from the patient-physician relationship. The reports illustrate the uncertainties of comparing a new agent to one already known to be active. One group of patients may consist of more rapid responders than another—that is, have patients who are not quite so sick as in another group—so a drug equal to the standard may really be no better than a placebo.

The statistical difficulties are severe, too. It has been claimed by statisticians that seven hundred subjects are necessary to avoid false conclusions about the efficacy of any new drug. Now that peptic ulcers are so readily treated by acid-ablating measures or by antibiotics, enlisting that many patients to compare one new drug with a placebo is not feasible. Gastroenterologists are so convinced that antibiotics will eliminate ulcers forever that the question may never arise.

It is easier to agree when controlled trials with placebos are not in order: when (1) death or disability may result without treatment, (2) available therapy is very effective, or (3) the experimental drug is already proven effective and the trial is intended only to give exact numbers to the benefit for marketing reasons.

Informed Consent

The ethics of clinical trials hang on the differences between patients and subjects. Many physicians feel like double agents when carrying out clinical studies on their patients, uncertain whether they are advancing their own interests or those of the patients. It may never be possible to procure from an acutely sick patient valid informed consent to any kind of therapeutic trial. The forty-year-old man in the cardiac intensive care unit finds it hard to refuse to participate in a study when his own doctor leans over the bedrail to ask for his cooperation.

Physician as Double Agent

More and more physicians were acting as double agents way before managed care. When a pharmaceutical firm pays a physician to run a controlled trial in a private office, the patients are almost never told about the financial arrangements, which are deemed not to be part of informed consent. It is no different for the assistant professor in a medical school who knows that promotion depends on publications; although he or she may not receive direct financial benefits from enrolling patients in studies, other benefits are forthcoming, such as secretarial help, travel, and other perquisites paid for from the commercial support to the laboratory or medical school. When federal agencies, like the National Institutes of Health (NIH), support similar studies, there are requirements to enroll a certain number of subjects in each study, and there are penalties for failing to achieve the appropriate "body count." In enrolling patients for studies, some academic physicians wonder whether they are considering their own welfare more than their patients'. The studies are important, and I have no quarrel with them; but any doubts could be resolved by disclosing all financial arrangements and any others to the patients enlisted.[3] Whether those volunteer patients should also be paid needs far more discussion. Currently, for reasons that escape me, it is held unethical for doctors to pay volunteers to participate in studies. There are many other ways in which physicians can be double agents; the financial rewards for doing less rather than more are still large in managed care contracts.

Natural History

The natural history of Crohn's disease, an inflammation of the intestines, underlines why controlled trials are so essential. The natural history of a disease can temper the doctor's enthusiasm for doing something and can highlight the benefits that come from self-help. "A patient sick enough to require treatment on an ambulatory basis can get better with no specific drug therapy," according to doctors at New York's Mt. Sinai Hospital. In one trial they reported improvement in 25–40 percent of the patients who received no treatment at all. More impressive, three-quarters of the patients in remission stayed well without specific maintenance therapy over the next year; two-thirds remained well for at least two years. Physicians used to know that many patients, even with Crohn's disease, get better on their own, without treatment. Patients in such studies have continuing physician support and enthusiasm, which may have a lot to do with their getting and staying well. That is what placebos and alternative medical approaches tell us. Unfortunately, physicians rarely recognize the healing powers of nature—or the passage of time.[4]

Managed care administrators may cavil at too many visits, and physicians may worry that they are not really doing anything in follow-up visits, but experienced clinicians have long suspected that continuing contact with patients with Crohn's disease—and many other diseases, for that matter—prevents trouble. Patients must realize this too, for a number of people with Crohn's disease have asked for another appointment. That kind of medical contact may provide whatever placebos also provide, without medication.

Placebos as Therapy

Pharmacologically inactive, placebos have been called "a chemical device for psychotherapy, . . . largely devoid of pharmacological properties." Shapiro's definition is more specific. He says a placebo is "any therapy (or that component of any therapy) that is deliberately used for its non-specific psychologic or psychophysiologic effect, or that is used for its presumed specific effect on a patient, symptom, or illness, but which, unknown to *patient and therapist*, is without specific activity for the condition being treated" (Shapiro 1964).

Others agree on the powerful psychological effects of "any therapeutic procedure . . . which is objectively without specific activity for the condition treated." Howard Brody adds that "a placebo is used . . . for its symbolic effect."

Therapeutic placebos relieve pain and the kinds of symptoms I described in Chapter 1. The responsible mechanisms may remain uncertain, but from the physician's standpoint, the medical intent is important even if one doctor's drug may be another's placebo. In evaluating the effect of placebos on disease, the physician's intent is important to definitions, if not to the patient, whose role in the placebo effect looms large.

Science and Intuition

Let me define *science* and *intuition* as I use those terms throughout this book. I will spend more time on intuition than science, which is so much part of our daily lives and thoughts that it has become almost a religion. *Science* is the process by which new knowledge is created; it gives objective knowledge that is quantitative and verifiable. The scientific method depends on observation, experimentation, and replication; therefore, science depends on sensory organs, especially the eyes, and on instruments that magnify and record what scientists can see.

Beyond experimentation and control, the scientific method requires verification by others. For Bertrand Russell, "Science is the attempt to discover by means of observation, and reasoning based upon it, first, particular facts about the world and then laws connecting facts with one another and (in fortunate cases) making it possible to predict future occurrences." He adds, "Science does not include art, or friendship, or various other valuable elements in life. . . . Science can tell us much about the means of realizing our desires, but it cannot say that one desire is preferable to another" (Russell 1935).

Intuition, in contrast, is what we know by immediate apprehension, at a glance, without conscious activity. I think of intuition as knowledge that is nonmeasurable and nonquantifiable. The *Oxford English Dictionary* defines intuition as "immediate knowledge. . . . The immediate apprehension of an object by the mind without the intervention of any reasoning process." The *Random House Dictionary* defines intuition as "direct perception of truth, fact, etc., independent of any reasoning process; immediate apprehension."

William Montague distinguishes intuition from science in his discussion of romantic love: "It would surely be a vain and preposterous undertaking to discover one's true sweetheart by accepting the authority of others, by using deductive reasoning and calculation, by cold-blooded empirical analysis of her perceivable qualities, or by considering the extent to which she might be a practical utility."

Henri Bergson depicts intuition and intelligence as pointing in opposite directions. I find his explication very helpful. Intelligence, he says, is the tool that science uses to deal with matter, with things and quantitative relations, whereas intuition is inward and immediate, providing a vision of reality: "The former toward inert matter, the latter toward life."

The theologian Martin Buber gives a rich interpretation of intuition: "We must develop in ourselves and in the next generation a gift which lives in man's inwardness as a Cinderella, one day to be a princess. Some call it intuition, but that is not a wholly unambiguous concept. I prefer the name 'imagining the real,' for in its essential being this gift is not a looking at the other, but a bold swinging, demanding the most intensive stirring of one's being, into the life of the other."

Bertrand Russell derides intuition, comparing it to "mysticism." "When a man of science tells us the result of an experiment, he also tells us how the experiment was performed; others can repeat it, and if the result is not confirmed it is not accepted as true. . . . The mystic himself may be certain that he knows, and has no need of scientific tests but those who are asked to accept his testimony will subject it to the same kind of scientific tests as those applied to men who say they have been to the North Pole. I cannot admit any method of arriving at truth except that of science, but in the realm of the emotions I do not deny the value of the experiences which have given rise to religion" (Russell 1935).

For the scientist, intuition can lead to serendipity. The prepared mind is able to grasp a new opportunity; it has what the neurobiologist calls hard-wired circuits, ready to go with the proper calcium influx. For one retired physician, H. R. Jacobs, musing over the discoveries that had come early in his career, intuition was the "welcome stranger . . . , essentially wild . . . , invisible, inaudible, and imponderable. It is not subject to scientific testing because it is not amenable to scientific procedures; certainly it cannot be summoned at will."

In a sense, then, as Bergson suggests, science deals with matter, and intuition with mind, those two hoary philosophical poles. Someone has suggested that matter pushes, whereas mind pulls—a nice distinction.

The knowledge of science is quantifiable; the knowledge of intuition is not. This is the difference between intelligence and emotion, or physics and poetry. Poetic imagination sometimes may prove as illuminating to medical practice as science, but in judging the claims of alternative medicine, science is required. If two claims are made for cure of a disease, one by a faith healer and the other by a mainstream investigator, both must be assessed on a scientific basis. As Russell says, "What I do wish to maintain—and it is here that the scientific attitude becomes imperative—is that insight, untested and unsupported, is an insufficient guarantee of truth, in spite of the fact that much of the most important truth is first suggested by its means. . . . Instinct, intuition, or insight is what first leads to the beliefs which subsequent reason confirms or confutes" (Russell 1935). I will have more to say about intuition and the romantic stream in Chapter 12.[5]

Physicians talk so much about "truth" and "facts" that it is worthwhile considering the *Oxford English Dictionary* definition of *fact* as "something that has really occurred or is actually the case . . . a particular truth known by actual observation or authentic testimony, as opposed to what is merely inferred." *Truth* is defined, synonymously, as "conformity with fact."

In this regard, let me note the contrast between Yale's law school and its medical school. It often struck me during the five years that I had an office at the law school that Yale lawyers seemed to regard the law as created, not discovered, and as changing over time. The case method was much used in classes: the facts of a case were ascertained, and discussion was voluble. Then the instructor would suggest, "But supposing the man had been a woman or . . . ," changing first one aspect of the case, then another. The ensuing decisions varied depending on the changes in the details.

In contrast, in Yale's medical school, as in most others, students are taught that facts are immutable, that scratching away to find them will bring out the truth, and that there really is only one truth. We need both points of view as we contemplate placebos and alternative medicine and the benefits that they may bring.

The fading repute of doctors today comes partly from a generally decreased respect for authority and partly from the physician's climb to riches; but it also comes from the awesome achievements of scientific medicine. When physicians could do little, they got credit for the occasional recovery, but now that so many patients can be cured of serious diseases, the doctor is blamed when recovery or relief is not quick. Death even seems like a disease that can be indefinitely put off. Moreover, modern physicians, imbued with notions of patient-physician equality, have little faith in themselves as therapeutic agents and run the risk of antagonizing their patients by a take-it-or-leave-it attitude. If the doctor doesn't seem to be trying to help, patients are entitled to get angry. Giving out pills used to be one way of showing that the doctor cared, but the growing availability of technology has turned diagnostic tests into more scientific reassurance, really a kind of placebo. I will suggest later that postmodern and alternative physicians may be changing all that.

Early Use of Placebos

In the past, physicians may have given placebos thinking they were giving active medicines. Early or primitive medicine is derided as only the history of the placebo, an assertion that highlights the devaluation of placebos in modern medicine and denies that hope helps. Plato and Aristotle turned to the physician and to medical methods for their model of philosophy, so they must have found some value in the profession. To ridicule medical history as merely the history of the placebo until modern times is to endorse the biomedical-mechanical model of disease and to ignore the caring role of the profession. The nonspecific benefits of advice about hygiene, nutrition, and even exercise may have contributed to what early physicians did for their patients.

Much of what early physicians achieved may have depended as much on patient-physician relationships as on time-tested remedies. It surely cannot have been only statistical quirks or the tendency of most things to pass for which physicians took credit. They did comfort, and their comforting helped. For many patients, that was enough, even when physicians gave harmful pills or potions in the faith that they would help. Too wide a disparagement of medical practices of the past seems ungenerous.

When Physicians Use Placebos

In Chapter 12, I consider why modern physicians have learned to avoid placebos. Most physicians have grown defensive about them, saying that their colleagues might use placebos but attributing their own therapeutic success to less personal factors.

I distinguish between belief and intent when physicians give placebos; some believe that they are giving an active drug, whereas others intend to give an inactive agent.[1] For the relief of pain, physicians usually try the weakest therapeutic agent first, aspirin or acetaminophen (Tylenol) before percocet, acetaminophen before codeine, codeine before morphine, and so forth. If modern physicians think of placebos at all, they consider them weak pain-relieving agents with few side effects, helpful for minor pains or anxiety but not for anything severe.

Physicians use placebos as a gift, challenge, or ransom.

The Placebo as a Gift

In the most generous mode, physicians give pills to relieve pain of uncertain origin or to treat a complaint that seems likely to have no objective explanation. Wisely wary of giving analgesics that might be addicting, they know that anxiety enhances the awareness of pain and that it may yield to the symbolic caress of a pill.

The Placebo as a Challenge

Sometimes physicians use placebos as a challenge, to prove to the patient and to themselves that the complaints are imaginary or exaggerated. In the waning years of this century, patients most likely to receive placebos as a challenge are those whose pain has no detectable origin. Placebos given in such an adversary mode are being misused: "See, if a sugar pill has helped you, your illness is all in your mind." Next in line are (1) postoperative patients who ask for pain relief or administer it to themselves longer than the staff thinks they should; (2) those who seem to be too dependent on narcotics to relieve chronic pain or discomfort; and (3) complainers, who are always asking for something and who remain unhappy.

Today's physicians prefer to prescribe an active placebo for nonspecific symptoms—that is, a medication known to be effective but not for the complaints to be treated—in the apparent hope that having given something that "works," the doctor can ascribe the symptoms to a real disease or to a physiological mechanism that has gone awry. Everyone is satisfied, and a confrontation with emotional issues is avoided, even if relief comes from symbolic rather than pharmacological effects. The H-2 blockers are probably the commonest agents now used in this manner because they reduce acid secretion and relieve the pain of peptic ulcer. Used like this, H-2 blockers fall into the category of active placebos, a matter amplified in Chapter 4. Now that they are freely available over the counter, physicians may have to look for some other elegant and equally harmless prescription.

The Placebo as a Ransom

To get rid of patients who have become too difficult and who complain all the time, physicians may turn to placebos as a sop, to deceive. Patients so pacified are then branded as crocks, a label that spares doctors and nurses from trying to help. In such circumstances, placebos tell the staff that the patient is beyond their concern: "We found that placebos were rarely prescribed—about one prescription per year per physician—but that, in almost every instance in which a placebo was prescribed, the physician and staff were having great difficulty relating to a particular patient. Physicians and nurses may need to prove that such difficult and unlikable patients are not really ill because they need to believe that they would never become so angry and frustrated with a genuinely ill person" (Goodwin).

Giving a placebo as a ransom is justified only when it is the first step in a genuine therapeutic approach.

The Physician: Healer or Conduit?

Placebos benefit patients regardless of the mood in which doctors prescribe them—that is one of their wonders. The intent of the physicians must be taken into account, but that is something we can judge only by what they know and what they tell us. Sophisticated physicians recognize that sometimes even an active drug is really a placebo, whereas more activist physicians, out of ignorance or innocence, may believe that their pills help by a specific pharmacological action.

The shared faith of physician and patient is always helpful, but to be a pure placebo, a drug must be considered inactive by the prescriber. Still, placebos work not only when they are given as a gift, challenge, or ransom but also when they are given in the mistaken belief that they are effective. Even though the placebo benefits only by virtue of the physician-patient relationship, the point is clear: the power of the placebo lies in the patient's response more than in the physician.

On the other hand, a National Institutes of Health study reaffirmed the importance of the doctor in enhancing the effectiveness of placebos. When clinicians expected their patients to improve more with one placebo than with another, the patients taking the preferred drug reported more pain relief than those taking the other. The question naturally arises, "Why is it deceitful to give a placebo if a large element of modern therapeutics is no better than placebo? Is the gullibility of a good-hearted doctor preferable to (and more ethical than) the skepticism of one whose prescription is pharmacologically inert, when the results are the same?" (Lancet)

When most medicines are prescribed, as they are today, with appar-

ent scientific rationale, physicians rely much less o[...]
therapeutic agents than on their prescriptions and proc[...]
too embarrassed to try to be a healer, and relegate any[...]
fictitious charisma. Antibiotics, not compassion, cure[...]
ulcers, they would say, and quite correctly. Yet the s[...]
tive medical practices in making patients feel better may be changing
this mindset.

One recurrent, if paradoxical, theme is that the more medical science does for disease, the less physicians do for patients. When hospitals became corporate enterprises with battalions of staff wielding high-technology devices against disease, individual physicians began to count for less and less. Even in their offices, physicians have come to rely increasingly on diagnostic and therapeutic technology, far more than on the comfort their personal skills could still assure. Even much-praised primary care practitioners have turned into triage officers or symphony conductors, sending patients to different kinds of specialists to find the cause of their trouble or coordinating the concerted search.

The new dispensation of managed care and HMOs has put a premium on time. Some years ago in my university clinic, making money was never an explicit consideration, and time was unbounded; now, seeing patients as rapidly as possible has become exquisitely important. HMOs have had to recognize the bewildered frustration of many patients whose psychosocial and emotional problems cannot be solved by medical manipulation and who have become "high-utilizers." Facing larger and larger numbers of complainers, HMOs are adopting group psychotherapeutic techniques to trim costs and are even turning to alternative practitioners as they rediscover the old psychosomatic models in which mind and body are seen as one. It is too early to tell whether such approaches will decrease the financial outlays of HMOs.[2]

Physicians in Hospitals

Reliance on therapeutic technology once characterized only university hospitals, but as thousands of physicians trained in technology moved out to community hospitals over the past forty years, the community hospitals came to resemble their university counterparts.

.en someone is dying," a friend in one such hospital remarked, they call for the priest to give last rites and the cardiologist to pass a Swan." During its heyday the Swan-Ganz catheter was inserted into almost every dying patient to measure the strength of the heart. Its use is far less ubiquitous today.

Although technological advances have vastly improved the prospect for many acute medical problems; family physicians have had little to do with such technology. Respirators, catheters, pacemakers, and other paraphernalia are lifesavers, but they require the expertise of an aco-lyte-technician or physician-specialist—a "hospitalist," as the latest jargon has it. Intensive care units (ICUs), coronary care units (CCUs), and a whole panoply of special interests have carved our hospitals into specialized duchies, each with its own boss and hierarchy. The power of the medical dukes is being challenged and weakened by the rise of managed care empires, however.

In spite of the current hoopla about family physicians, most big hospitals make little room for general physicians who take care of patients without specific technical skills. Increasingly, even specialists turn their critically sick patients over to hospitalists and their teams. The new arrangements limit the physicians' view of what they do even as managed care administrators in a lust for cost cutting urge family doctors to do more than they have been trained to do.[3] A few years after training, even cardiologists, the prototypical specialists, are often at a loss to deal with the ever changing apparatus, so quickly do new discoveries make medical skills obsolete. An earnest physician might once have sat some hours by the bed of a patient with a heart attack watching for arrhythmia or another doleful blow. Now such patients are quickly turned over to the video monitors in the CCU, to nurses, resident physicians, and CCU specialists. That is good for the patients, but the progress of medicine has led to skepticism about what any individual physician can do. Yet the more powerless the individual doctors feel, the louder their patients clamor for family physicians to guide and befriend them.

Turning family physicians into gatekeepers also makes doctors double agents. They serve the economic welfare of the HMO as much as the patient in front of them, and that will surely lead to trouble.

Hospital-based physicians can be more than simple conduits of power if they give old-fashioned encouragement. Years ago, anesthetists at the Massachusetts General Hospital studied two groups of patients undergoing elective operations. One group was given no specific information about postoperative pain; the other was told what to expect and how to allay such pain. "The presentation was given in a manner of enthusiasm and confidence; the patients were not informed that we were conducting a study. The surgeons, not knowing which patients were receiving special care, continued their practices as usual." The patients given special advice required half the usual amount of narcotics in the postoperative period. "The anesthetist who understands his patient and who believes that each patient is 'his' patient ceases to be merely a clever technician in the operating room" (Egbert). Presumably anyone, not only a physician, could help to reduce the amount of narcotics required; but the point remains that physicians can still do a lot for their patients if they keep them informed enough to help themselves.[4]

Current wisdom holds that more family practitioners are needed because they will be less expensive than subspecialists. But they are needed for the worried well, who are not sick enough to need the attention that hospitals give. Everyone is pushing for more family doctors. It is hard for me to believe that changing that balance will improve medical care for the very sick. Indeed, evidence continues to show that family doctors and general internists do not treat patients with cardiac problems anywhere near as well as cardiologists do, and the same is true for patients with stroke, AIDS, and other serious diseases. That commonsense idea is being lost in the rush to primary care.

Physicians in Offices

For the past few years, the only patients likely to be admitted to a hospital have been those with a potentially perilous disease. That battlefield against death is no longer the best place for most physicians to get their training for future practice in offices or in outpatient clinics, where diseases are chronic and complaints often without detectable origin. Estimates of the frequency of emotional factors in outpatients vary enormously, depending on what the observer defines as functional disease. For Richard Cabot at the Massachusetts General Hospital in 1904, almost half the patients coming to the medical clinic had functional diseases, by which he meant constipation, dyspepsia, debility, apprehension, and the like. Sixty years later, studies in the same hospital suggested that in more than 80 percent of the patients psychological distress was the major impetus for attendance at the medical clinic. Psychological distress was a common factor in the decision to get help, something any practitioner awakened in the middle of the night could have told them without a study.

Many complaints seen in office and clinic have no detectable biological origin, even though most mainstream physicians begin with the opposite assumption in the fear of missing something in a patient who is really sick. Doctors would rather err in thinking that patients have a disease when they do not than err in thinking that patients are well when they are really sick. Doctors take the safer course partly to avoid lawsuits, now a well-known reason why costs have climbed so high. If doctors did not have to practice defensive medicine, they might rely more than they now do on relieving symptoms.

It is sad to remark how even in their offices many physicians now see themselves as simple conduits of the powerful forces of technology and their main job as helping patients make their own choices. In part, that is a consequence of the movement to make patients equal partners with doctors. Aging physicians, a little slow to keep up with the latest wrinkle, used to stay behind their office desk, where they treated other aging people with chronic disorders, and they turned patients with acute problems over to younger colleagues. Now, however, those kind physicians have come under attack as parentalistic, and what they before took as their duty is now seen as reprehensibly authoritarian. Practicing physicians do not always understand modern technology—and may not need to—but their penchant for advice giving has also come under criticism. It sometimes seems that physicians have little left to feel good about.

Controlled clinical trials have contributed to this conviction that the physician is simply a conduit of pills and procedures. Holding all physicians equal in a trial implicitly suggests that the specific physician does not matter, that they are all the same.

Similarly, managed care, with its growing reliance on so-called game plans and disease management to define quality, treats all physicians and other health care providers as modules, paying little attention to varying skills or knowledge or abilities of individual doctors.[5]

Doctors' Personal Qualities

Manual dexterity varies, making one surgeon more skilled than another. Pattern recognition, which is the ability to interpret X-rays and other images, depends on more than training. Only psychiatrists explicitly confess that the ability to heal may also vary from one physician to another.

Surely there is as much variation in physicians as in patients. In the trials of ulcer therapy discussed earlier, physicians evoked different placebo responses, which is to say that their healing capacities varied, and these rates remained consistent over the years. The personal qualities of physicians have a large role in the placebo response, even though most ulcer researchers take it for granted that only the characteristics of the crater and the medication influence healing. We can measure the dimensions of the ulcer, but we should not ignore the doctor who treats it any more than we ignore the patient who has the ulcer. An angry doctor, or one hostile or cold, may well slow the healing process or lessen the placebo response.

The new lamentable controls in American medicine have brought growing resentment on the part of physicians. Modern doctors are already driven by training to prove—that is, to see—by technological means what is wrong with the patient; now managed care plans have made doctors into employees and allow them little time to listen to their patients, engendering a frustration that may well make the harried physicians more grudgingly curt in their treatment of patients. The placebo effect comes in part from the authority of physicians and the esteem in which they are held; if decisions must be cleared by faraway third-party clerks who search on a video screen for suitable rules and incantations, physicians will feel ever more like the interchangeable units that they are becoming. I fear for their patients.

Charismatic Healing

These days, any benefit from the laying on of hands is considered embarrassing to physicians and demeaning to patients. For that reason, prescribing placebos makes many physicians feel guilty at their nonscientific attitude. My colleague Robert Burt comments: "The rigor with which the placebo effect must be eliminated before any medical intervention can be viewed as efficacious points to two critical aspects of contemporary physicians' views of themselves: first, that the magical 'laying on of hands' which had such prominence in earlier physicians' views of their calling is now widely seen as inconsistent with the highest aspiration of medical practice. . . . A physician who aspires to scientific objectivity can properly assert that, insofar as the efficacy of his therapy depends on his personal will, he has transgressed the norms of his profession."

The healing power of charismatic medicine demands clinical trials, which are hard to arrange. A definition of charisma is pertinent here, for the word has achieved a considerable popularity in medical circles. The Oxford English Dictionary defines charisma as "a free gift or favour specially vouchsafed by God; a grace, a talent." In more secular medical circles, charismatic healing usually refers to the personal authority of the physician and any benefit that may bring.

Self-Image

How much physicians vary in their charismatic healing, and why, needs contemplation. How much does the physicians' image of themselves affect their patients and their therapeutic effectiveness? The model or the metaphor that doctors choose for their calling is important: physicians who think of themselves as fathers or mothers will act differently from those who think of themselves as soldiers fighting disease, and consequently they will have a different relationship with their patients.

Physicians who see themselves as scientists searching out the facts will find that it is their duty to be thoroughly objective, whereas those who think of themselves as detectives will have a different view of their duty. Clinical research has been compared to the Olympics, a view of medicine as sport that implies a certain competitiveness, as anyone who has watched a college football game will appreciate. The burst of energy with which Yale and Harvard vie in the final seconds suggests how the metaphor of the Olympics might carry over into the diagnostic process as an attempt to effect on the body of the patient the one-in-a-hundred victory. The physician who was a hockey player in college will bring different skills and viewpoints to the medical enterprise than one who was a dancer, a poet, or even a long-distance runner. That women, compared with men, might bring differing attitudes to medicine once seemed likely, but the changes so far have been hard for me to find.[6]

Other models have served in other cultures. For example, in Chinese medicine, so Jing-Bao Nie tells us, *The Emperor's Medical Classic* declares that, like a good general who tries to avert war, a good doctor treats disease by preventing it, using medical procedures only at a last resort, to minimize side effects. Although Western medicine also has its military metaphors, the emphasis on prevention should appeal to the postmodern clinician in our Sinophilic times.

Physicians who see themselves as powerless conduits and who see placebos as useless may prescribe placebos only as a challenge, no matter how comforting they want to be. We physicians cannot avoid the placebo effect, but we can make it helpful or destructive depending on our attitude.

Physicians as Active Agents

The idea that physicians help their patients only with pills and procedures and not with their advice and comfort has been growing since modern medicine began to focus on disease rather than on patients. In 1938, a well-known physician of the time, W. B. Houston, considered all the medicines up to his time placebos that reinforced words of cheer and comfort. Of earlier physicians he said, approvingly: "Their learning was a learning in how to deal with men. Their skill was a skill in dealing with the emotions of men. They themselves were the therapeutic agents by which cures were effected. . . . The history of medicine is a history of the dynamic power of the relationship between doctor and patient."

The psychobiological implications of disease seemed so important to him that he wanted to strengthen physicians' faith in themselves; the patient was only the passive clay for the physician to mold: "The faith that heals must have deep roots in the personality of the healer." He asked, "How can the doctor himself, as a therapeutic agent, be refined and polished to make of him a more potent agent?" That question still needs to be asked today. He added, "One cannot advance against the disorders in the emotional sphere by mere reasoning."

A while back, a physician received a telephone call from a friend in another city, who told him that he had had a heart attack and was confused by various alternatives. Advice duly having been offered and accepted, the friend said, "You know, that is why I called. I know you don't know a damned thing about the heart, but I knew you would have an opinion and would state it directly and forcefully, and that makes me feel much better." Part of the charismatic grace must lie in the merging of physician and patient, which may bring as much to the doctor as to the patient. As Burt put it: "Many doctors and patients do clearly conceive themselves as psychologically merged in their dealings. . . . The patient's pain will vanish when he conceives himself and the world as one." Giving an honest placebo joins doctor and patient in a confession that none of us knows how healing comes, even if we understand the power of a close patient-physician relationship. I discuss transference and countertransference, so important in this regard, in Chapter 12.

Physicians may need more faith in themselves, but an even greater danger lies in their having too high an opinion of their abilities. Giving a placebo as a magic potion without thinking about what he or she is doing might dangerously inflate the physician's self-image if the placebo works.

As medical practice grows more scientific, expanding its already vast array of technical devices, as medical science becomes better at treating organic disease, physicians have trouble coming to terms with complaints that have no objective counterpart: pain with no apparent cause, symptoms that appear and vanish inexplicably and the like. They are criticized for being cold and uninterested because their favorite techniques are those of technology and the laboratory.

Most *definitions of a placebo* focus on what it does; and the more precisely that can be measured, the better. To modern physicians, objective evidence, when quantified, is preferable to a subjective report. That is why truth in medicine has moved from patients and what they say to physicians and what they find. For the physician-scientist, a placebo is an inert substance that makes no detectable change in what instruments can measure, regardless of whether it changes what the patient feels and reports.

Milk, once the sovereign remedy for ulcer pain, offers a good example of how objective data have displaced subjective reports. For many years milk was the staple of the ulcer diet, relieving dyspepsia and pain to general satisfaction. When laboratory studies showed that milk did not reduce gastric acid but actually increased it, physicians began warning patients against milk and in its stead advised large amounts of antacids to neutralize stomach acid. Very few physicians could ever recall anyone whose dyspepsia worsened because of drinking milk, but an unwanted effect had been shown in the laboratory, so milk was banished from therapy. Today the doctor who tells a patient to take milk for dyspepsia is deemed invincibly ignorant, even though many people still find quick and cheap relief from a glass of milk.[1]

Studies of exorphins and prostaglandins offered some support for clinical impressions. Milk and similar foods, when digested by gastric juice mixtures, are turned into amino acids and polypeptides, which in turn act like endorphin pain relievers. Moreover, phospholipids of milk are surface-protecting agents. The details are not important, for my point is not to defend milk or dietary therapy when antibiotics and antacid agents are so much more effective, but to show how reports of pain relief are disparaged as subjective, less convincing than more objective laboratory evidence.

Incidentally, now that many foods are viewed as medication, or at least as positively good or bad for health, I have to confess to a degree of skepticism about so-called nutriceuticals, foods taken as medicine, for their therapeutic or preventive effects. I view food as pleasure, not medicine, and although some foods may be bad for some people when taken in excess, moderation in all things still makes sense, from food to exercise.

If I give a pill to a patient in distress and he or she is relieved, something has happened. If the same pill relieves pain in other patients, I can claim that it has an effect, even if I have not looked for changes in the brain by magnetic resonance imaging (MRI) or positron emission tomography (PET) scan, both of which show thoughts in "living color." To another patient in distress I can then say, quite truthfully, "This pill has helped others, and I hope that it will help you, even if I don't understand how it works." But not all doctors agree on the value or ethics of such prescriptions.

Pure and Impure Placebos

The difference between a pure and an impure placebo is fundamental. A pure placebo should be completely inert; composed of something like starch or sugar, it is given only for its psychological benefit. Any physiological changes because of that symbolic effect are taken into consideration only by behavioral scientists. Unfortunately, as I remarked earlier, what is deemed inactive at one time may prove to have physiological effects later. Lactose pills, so beloved as an inactive placebo by an earlier generation of investigators, turned out to have gastrointestinal side effects and are not used as placebos any longer.

An impure placebo has a known pharmacological effect irrelevant to the clinical problem for which it is prescribed. Into this category fall a vast array of mildly active agents or injections: many antispasmodic agents, multivitamins, and antibiotics. Other substances, like H-2 blockers, fall into this category when not used for a specific indication; they carry enough pharmacological consequences that physicians can console themselves with the hope that the drug might work, even if not on the symptom under treatment. "If nothing else is available, a doctor who believes he has nothing to prescribe may be unwilling to prescribe a placebo and may thereby also eliminate himself as a therapeutic agent. . . . A safe pharmaceutical agent, with a reasonable rationale for usage, may sometimes be desirable even if some of its results are not substantially better than those of placebo" (Feinstein).

An impure placebo that brings side effects like the dry mouth of antispasmodic agents may earn an enhanced placebo effect, its recipient surmising that if the drug is strong enough to dry the mouth, it must be doing some good elsewhere. From such considerations, presumably, came the bitter tonics and pretty pills of the old pharmacopoeia. In general, however, impure placebos may do as much harm as good, given the possibility of side effects. On the other hand, an active placebo may prove to be a stronger defense against a malpractice suit than an inactive one.

Over-the-counter (OTC) drugs must have a large placebo effect because of the context in which they are taken and the persuasive advertising that encourages expectations. In reviewing the effectiveness of those drugs, the FDA winnowed many out of the market, leaving only those deemed safe and effective. When directions are followed, some could represent unique and harmless combinations of active agents whose effect is augmented by advertising, custom, and expectation. Indeed, I once jocularly suggested that the FDA encourage the marketing of some such agents on the thesis that if they worked, they could be taken readily OTC, but nobody liked my idea.

Can you give yourself a placebo? To explain why you can, a popular writer, Morton Hunt, has invoked the willing suspension of disbelief. We can talk ourselves into hope, and do so every day. Hunt maintains that this is self-suggestion, not self-deception, and I suppose it is not very different from such measures as the relaxation response that Herbert Benson has described. Sick doctors often go to some length to find the "best" doctor, and only when they are satisfied with their choice do they relax and take advice. That search, too, may offer some kind of placebo effect.

Procedures as Placebos

A placebo does not have to be a pill. An injection, an operation, even a diagnostic procedure like an endoscopy, can work as a placebo. Modern diagnostic procedures, still lavishly paid for, are so welcomed with enthusiasm by physician and patient alike that they may be placebos and are so credited by many physicians. Even if the procedure is being done to reassure, its effect is still that of a placebo.

Injections

Behavioral responses play a big role in the placebo response to injections. Placebo injections may relieve pain better than pills because they require someone else to give the shot. Any injection is loaded with behavioral cues, depending on how often the patient has had injections before, for what reason, and with what previous benefit. Something penetrating the skin and hurting a little must evoke stronger physiological mechanisms, whatever they may be, than simply taking a pill, however sacramental the circumstances.

Mack Lipkin long ago described using an arcane electric apparatus as a placebo in patients with painful fingers and joints. He did not turn on the current, just clicked the dials. Every patient reported some improvement, and in six the results were excellent. "Suggestion was undoubtedly responsible for the result in these," Lipkin concluded.[2]

Operations

Henry Beecher first emphasized that surgery could evoke a placebo effect and cautioned against accepting the benefit of any new operation until properly designed tests ruled out the bias of the patient or the surgeon. Edzard Ernst has suggested that any invasive procedure that involves the patient's body, even one as meek as acupuncture, sweeps the patient up in a powerful placebo effect, far stronger than any drugs taken by mouth. As I have already suggested, that may be why, as placebos, injections sometimes seem more helpful than pills.

These days it would be highly unethical, even with informed consent, to carry out a sham operation, to lead the patient to believe that something has been done when it has not. Yet in the 1950s just such a trial was carried out to test internal mammary artery ligation, an operation believed to help angina pectoris by increasing blood flow to the heart. The surgeons incised the skin under local anesthesia in all patients, but that is all they did in half the patients. The results were surprising at the time: *all* subjects reported a decreased need for nitroglycerin and increased exercise tolerance.

Later, another operation on the same artery to enhance blood flow to the heart brought an 85 percent improvement rate. That procedure was finally given up, but not before "10,000 to 15,000 operations were performed, with an average operative mortality of approximately 5%." Herbert Benson, who has gone on to elevate the placebo response to the effect of "remembered wellness," comments on the objective changes recorded in these studies: "increased exercise tolerance, reduced nitroglycerin usage, and improved electrocardiographic results. . . . Patient and physician belief in the efficacy of the therapy and a continuously strong physician-patient relationship should maintain the effects for long periods." Ironically, the same artery is now the one used to supply a conduit to the heart in the current bypass procedure.

In the 1980s, bypass operations relieved the chest pain of heart trouble much better than medical treatment did, but in other respects people who received only medical treatment lived just as long as those who had undergone an operation, and they were just as likely to return to work. In other words, the main benefit of cardiac surgery at that time seemed to be relief of pain. Techniques have much improved since then, and the overall outlook is better, but cardiologists usually ascribe pain relief after an operation to surgical interruption of pain fibers, as well as to the more generous supply of blood vessels to the heart muscle.

Not many are willing to consider that the operation might also bring a placebo benefit. Yet just looking at the very impressive scar on your chest, knowing that a surgeon has had your heart in his or her hands and that an operation to improve the blood supply has been carried out, surely must give some push to hope, if not to endorphin levels. That scar over the heart must be an important reminder of relief. I underwent a bypass operation for anginal pain a few years ago to prevent heart damage, and I have no pain when I walk, but I do not expect to live any longer than if I had taken only medication. Still, I am very grateful for that pain relief regardless of how much may be placebic. More than 500,000 such operations were done in 1996 alone, with a very low mortality rate.

New operations to relieve abdominal pains come along without end; they are used for a few years, then reevaluated and often abandoned. This sequence is particularly true for operations planned to deal with discoveries by the newest diagnostic devices. Their findings are wrenched into place as an explanation for abdominal pain, then advanced as a universal explanation. Doctors eradicate the abnormality by operation or by drugs until, after some years, it becomes clear that the reported abnormality is only an unoffending normal variant, not as important as it had seemed. Such operations are not successful for very long. Many explanations for abdominal pain have been advanced over the years, although neither the diagnostic procedure nor the operation designed to remove what it has uncovered has been credited with a placebo effect.

A good example is offered by the patient—sadly, often a woman—with abdominal pain of uncertain cause, a common and challenging phenomenon.[3] In the 1950s, when X-ray studies of the stomach became more sophisticated, "antral pyloric mucosal prolapse" was first detected at fluoroscopy. Found in young women with abdominal pain (because more women than men came to be X-rayed), it was deemed the cause of abdominal pain, nausea, and belching. Once a lesion is seen, physicians have an irresistible temptation to remove or fix it, so several hundred women underwent operations to remove the bottom part of the stomach or to tighten up the supposed prolapse. The operation proved worthless after a few years and was abandoned.

Some time later, X-ray techniques to visualize the blood vessels of the body came into vogue; that led to the delineation of "celiac axis stenosis" as the culprit in some women with otherwise unexplained abdominal pain. After quite a few blood vessels had been loosened up with only short-term benefit, the operation and the concept were largely abandoned. More recently, radioactive techniques have measured how quickly the stomach empties itself of food. As might have been expected, some stomachs empty faster than others, but now the same kind of patients who a few years ago stood accused of celiac axis stenosis or antral mucosal prolapse are told that they have delayed gastric emptying. Such patients take drugs to speed up their sluggish emptying, and when that does not work, they run the risk of an operative procedure to promote emptying. That, too, will probably prove to be just another in a long series of ill-conceived notions to fix a working body part, no more effective than attempts in the 1920s to tie down a floating kidney or to restore a mobile cecum to its normal resting place in the abdominal cavity.

Nausea is a very common complaint. It may arise from medication or, very rarely, from something as serious as a brain tumor, but in otherwise healthy people it mostly has no discoverable cause. Everyone is nauseated by the smell of vomit; study at that time would doubtless find gastric motility delayed as a reflection of that nausea. Nausea can also come from disgust ("It makes me sick to my stomach"), for we humans react to metaphors with our bodies as well as our minds. Modern doctors dislike that idea.

Bouginage

Many lesser procedures act as placebos. Stretching the esophagus by a balloon or a tube relieves the chest pain of esophageal spasm because, most gastroenterologists believe, it renders the gullet incapable of quite such fierce contractions. That may not be the whole story. Some Navy physicians studied the response of patients to thin and thick tubes, called bougies. As a placebo, they inserted a thin bougie, far too narrow to stretch the esophagus. The active treatment involved dilation with a much thicker bougie because of what they took to be its real therapeutic potential. They found no difference between the effects of the thin and fat bougies, either on chest pain or on ease of swallowing. All patients had an impressive decrease in the severity of chest pain, leading the physicians to conclude that one mechanism might have been a placebo effect from the close physician-patient interaction.

Why such operations help patients for even a short while is what this book is about. Changed perception, postoperative pain, the attentive care the patient receives after surgery, the mystery of the operation itself, and, finally, the symbolic value of the scar—all these contribute. The history of modern medicine is replete with such examples. Operations may work as placebos because of the enormous metabolic changes that they engender: sooner or later, when the right hormones or neurotransmitters can be measured, physicians will rejoice at the explanation and only then recognize that some such operations are arduous placebos.

Such observations confirm that operations have a placebo effect no different from that of pills. Long an explorer of the placebo effect, Herbert Benson has commented that "this remarkable efficacy should not be disregarded or ridiculed. After all, unlike most other forms of therapy, the placebo effect has withstood the test of time and continues to be safe and inexpensive." He emphasizes the importance of communicating confidence in the therapy but, despite fear that it might be deceptive to appear too confident, sensibly calls for reasonable enthusiasm to increase the placebo effect.

Alternative Medicine

Many procedures used by mainstream medicine are no better than, or act as, placebos. That is, they relieve pain or foreboding or anxiety by their symbolic meaning, or they enhance the effect of some other agent or procedure. With only a small leap of faith we can extend that idea to alternative medicine and the whole field of complementary practices, from acupuncture to exercise.[4]

Patients are more important than their diseases. They
play the leading role in the placebo drama, for not
only their diseases but their expectations of pills or
procedures, their reactions to disease and doctor,
their very outlook on life, influence what placebos
can do. *Webster's Dictionary* used to define a patient
as "one that suffers, endures, or is victimized."
A more modern definition (*Random House*) calls a
patient "a person who is under medical care or
treatment." The *Oxford English Dictionary* also defines
a patient as "a sufferer . . . under medical treatment." The incorporation of suffering in
patienthood may seem old-fashioned, but it is
very appropriate.

chapter five

The

Patient

and the

Disease

Pharmacology

and Faith

Being a Patient Versus Being Sick

Someone who is sick becomes a patient when
he or she looks for help. Patients and physicians
have different purposes: patients want to talk
about their complaints, whereas physicians need
to turn the symptoms into a problem that they can
treat. The dialogue is inherently unequal: doctors
quickly take control because patients need help
and know less than the physicians about what may
be wrong, and they are worried about the outcome. What is common for physicians is far more
unusual for patients.

Doctors once made house calls, but now
patients go to doctors in offices and clinics. If a
secretary has not already given the patient who
comes to the doctor's office a checklist of symptoms
on computer, the physician has questions at the
ready. The patient is usually unfamiliar with what
will happen. Silence can be misinterpreted by
either one. Here is how one doctor, a psychiatrist,

describes the interview. "The physician interrogates the patient, who must be able to understand the questions, ask them of himself, and then report back accurately the answers. . . . Medical examining, with its heavy emphasis on questions, makes the sharpest subject-object differentiation. . . . Typically, I question you . . . we can change our language by changing our distance, just as we can change our distance by changing our language" (Havens).

What doctors expect from patients has changed a lot. Formerly, the ideal patient was passive, compliant, and dependent on the physician as "captain of the ship," but now doctors are urged to regard patients as partners, equal except in specific knowledge. In an attempt to create equality, the very term *patient* has been replaced successively by *consumer*, *client*, and, in some hospitals now, by *guest*, all reflecting new modes of thinking about medical practice. Patients are now regarded as commodities or units that can be bought or sold. More and more, we hear managed-care people refer to patients as covered lives or even as work products.

Patients come in as many varieties as physicians, even if in what follows I write about *the* patient. Each person has a different idea of what it means to be sick and varying expectations of a physician. Older doctors of the modern type like to be captain of the ship—the fading metaphor has been traced to Plato. Very few see themselves as agents of their patients. Yet to some patients, doctors differ very little from tailors, furniture polishers, or teachers; they are paid to do a specific job and no more. Not everyone wants to be prodded and pushed in every area of life and health by a physician. Past experiences with doctors are probably most important in determining how close a therapeutic connection people want. Family environment, nurture, all those factors that make each of us unique, influence what patients want, just as anticipation determines patients' responses to placebos.

The differences in how patients are regarded boil down to the difference between a patient and a case. A *patient* is a person who is sick and who feels bad, whereas a *case* is the record of the course of a disease in a person. The case tells of the disease as an entity, not the life of the patient. Yet the physician who looks at the biomedical case alone will miss most of illness. "One who reduces medical problems to physical factors concentrates on genes, biochemistry, physiology, and disease entities . . . personal concerns, including those of illness, are likely to be judged as incidental 'surface phenomena.' . . . Suffering, functioning, and level and quality of adaptation are excluded. . . . One who emphasizes the interconnections between biological, psychological, and social factors will judge individuals holistically" (Fabrega).

I commented earlier that modern doctors are keener on telling the truth than on helping the patient. Telling the truth bolsters the doctor's good opinion of his or her own uprightness, but it is unlikely to help a patient in a calamity. That may sound parentalistic, but the parental role is not always as bad as advertised, for sick patients need advice. Some academic discussions of patient equality pay too little attention to the distant protests of patients who look for relief before knowledge.

Recent immigrants from the country of faith healers, modern physicians know how to treat the structural defects of organic disease, but they cannot hear what is not spoken, and may not listen to what is said. Patients, on the other hand, are worried about what may come, and are more likely to ask, "Is this serious?" Those who have pain for which there is no readily apparent physical basis will get neither rest nor counsel nor reassurance until the physician has exhausted all diagnostic studies and them as well.

Many people do want to know exactly what is wrong; in tracing the rising costs of medical care, economists now blame patients as much as physicians. In the days before medical rationing, told that a given test had a one-in-a-hundred chance of detecting an abnormality, people usually chose to have it "to be sure." Even in cocktail party conversations, most laypeople want every new symptom meticulously traced to its origin, rather than simply accepting symptomatic relief. That betrays an excessive faith in what physicians can do.

Pain

Patients are relieved of pain and discomfort by placebos so often that one might expect something good to be said of placebos. But praise for placebos is very rare these days—except from the few who have carefully studied what they can do. "Placebos can be more powerful than, and reverse the action of, potent active drugs. The incidence of placebo reactions approaches 100% in some studies. Placebos can have profound effects on organic illnesses, including incurable malignancies. Placebos can often mimic the effects of active drugs" (Shapiro 1960). Widely held views like this usually do not distinguish the patient's response from improvement in the disease itself and so overestimate what placebos can do. The relief that placebos may bring has been obscured by uncritically rapturous claims. People are helped, and complaints are relieved, but I find no convincing evidence that diseases are changed for better or worse.

To be sure, people die of fright, of voodoo or hexing, of anxiety, and even of heartbreak. Such well-documented events are ascribed to heart irregularities, electrolyte imbalance, and other disturbances, but evidence that diseases like cancer or heart disease have disappeared or improved after any placebo is hard to find.[1]

Acute and Chronic Pain

There is a difference between disease and the reaction to it. If I hit my thumb with a hammer, the pain is in my thumb—or in my head—but if it is bad enough, I may hop around yelling, "Oh, oh!" or worse. My reaction to the pain, which is in my brain, may prove more impressive than the injury to my thumb and the stimulation of my C-fibers. My jumping around may in fact be helpful, for new evidence suggests that any motor activity diminishes pain perception through changes in brain mechanisms.

The middle-aged man with new indigestion may ignore it or take some proprietary remedy; if it does not go away, he will worry about having cancer until anxiety, more than pain, drives him to the doctor. Just deciding to see a physician may make him begin to feel better. Every physician has heard patients say, "You know, Doctor, ever since I made the appointment, I have felt well. I don't know why I'm here, but I thought I should come anyway." The physician's secretary or the telephone company could claim credit for spontaneous relief, but it is more likely due to the connection established with the physician. Most problems go away on their own, and patients make appointments when they feel the worst, just before the trouble begins to wane. Such natural waxing and waning accounts for more than a few of the triumphs of placebos and physicians, whether mainstream or alternative. But when enigmatic pain becomes chronic, it turns into a disease or at least is given some name like chronic pain syndrome.

Is the pain in your stomach or in your head? If your doctor says that you are fine, your dyspepsia may disappear because of reassurance or medication or because it was going away anyway. On the other hand, if the doctor looks grave and orders more tests, you will surely be more attentive to your digestion. If the physician warns, "Take this prescription for the next ten days, but be careful, because it has side effects," you may have even more to worry about. Hope or the pills can make you feel better while anxiety—thinking about that cancer—makes you worse. The disease and the patient form half the equation of which physicians and their therapy make up the other.

Pain and Suffering

Pain comes in for more attention in Chapter 7, but a few words are pertinent here. Suffering can come from pain but also from fear. As F. S. Fitzgerald writes, "Of course all life is a process of breaking down. . . . There is another sort of blow that comes from within—that you don't feel until it's too late to do anything about it, until you realize with finality that in some regard you will never be as good a man again."

Doctors try to distinguish between pain and the suffering it brings; pain from a known source can be borne with far more equanimity than pain of unknown origin. That is why studies of pain relief in a laboratory have so little practical import; a subject bearing pain inflicted by an investigator has quite a different reaction from that of the patient with belly pain no one understands. "Patients can writhe in pain from kidney stones and by their own admission not be suffering, because they 'know what it is'; they may also report considerable suffering from apparently minor discomfort when they do not know its source" (Cassell 1982).

Suffering comes from pain when people feel overwhelmed by the fear that they will never be the same again. Eric Cassell adds a clue to how placebos might work: "Recovery from suffering often involves help, as though people who have lost parts of themselves can be sustained by the personhood of others until their own recovers. This is one of the latent functions of the physicians: to lend strength. A group too may lend strength."

Disease and Illness

In a discussion of psychopathology, Andrew Sims takes disease to be identical with illness, as indeed someone studying the products of a disordered mind would have to do. The World Health Organization defines *health* as requiring "total well-being." What doctors treat and statistical variations from the norm that carry biological disadvantages are called *disease*. Doctors who treat the whole patient still must separate organic from functional disorders.

Organic Versus Functional Disorders

Physicians rarely think about exactly what they mean by *disease*. For most, the definition in the *Oxford English Dictionary* will suffice: "a condition of the body, or some part or organ of the body, in which its functions are disturbed or deranged; a morbid physical condition; . . . a departure from the state of health especially when caused by structural change." *Disorder* is "usually a weaker term than disease, and not implying structural change." Seeing and touching are a doctor's favorite diagnostic senses, the eyes and the fingers the oldest diagnostic tools. I will use the term *disease* as it is generally understood by physicians: whatever the clinician can detect with tools like X-rays and endoscopes in a person with a complaint. Silent disease is another matter, which involves value judgments.

Definition is not always that precise: function reflects structure, perhaps even at the level of the twists and turns of amino acids or electrical forces. "Form follows function," the Bauhaus architects used to say. Modern physicians are pragmatists, defining disease as what they can detect morphologically, biochemically, and now functionally.

Modern genetics is so entrancing because it shows form and function at their most elemental. DNA makes the code, RNA transmits it, but a change in the curve or order of an amino acid changes the message— and the person. The genetic code is metaphorically an alphabet: a d-o-g is not a g-o-d. That is why postmodern physicians have begun to recognize molecular perturbations as disease.

To call a disease "functional" in medical practice is another matter. Clinical experience for a very long time now has depended on the "anatomo-clinical gaze"; on what can be seen. Functional diseases, those complaints that we call illness, for which no structural derangements provide an explanation, somehow seem unreal to physicians. Irritable bowel, to be discussed shortly, provides an example of the blurred border between diseases, functional disorders, and illness. That personal response to disease called *illness* is determined by character, culture, and the way the problem is regarded by society; illness includes all the undesirable accompaniments of the disease, not least its effect on the family and on daily life, all of which involve value judgments, as persons with AIDS have found out.

Illness is what patients feel, regardless of their disease. Leon Eisenberg put it flatly: "Patients suffer 'illnesses'; physicians diagnose and treat diseases" (1977). Patients are sometimes loath to intrude on this division. A sociologist with Parkinsonism, M. Lefton, writes, "I think of the many times I have left my doctor's office taking with me the non-medical trials and tribulations that are not his concern as a professional specialist. To worry about what I worry about could severely handicap his practice as a neurologist." What a sad commentary on modern medicine.[2]

Attribution

What someone thinks has caused his or her trouble is very important to its relief. What sociologists call *attribution* is likely to reflect a group's ideas: today exercise and nutrition seem more important to the American public than emotion or even stress in causing disease. Susan Sontag reminds us that tuberculosis was romanticized as a disease of passion, as the ravages of frustration, "romantic agony," before its cause was known.

Self-Image

One's place in society determines how serious an illness appears. The professional tennis player will fear pain in the elbow more than a lawyer does. The young lawyer with Menière's disease may have scarring in his ear, but he is not dizzy when he asks questions in court. The teacher with ulcerative colitis may ignore her scarred and shriveled colon three months out of four, especially when she plays competitive tennis. When I was sick a few years ago, I worried about dying but even more about losing my memory. An athlete would feel worse about a stiff neck than I might.

Physicians who look at disease on the reductionist model will ignore the social and cultural problems that contribute to the illness, whereas physicians who take them into account are likely to order fewer tests and not pursue the cause of every complaint.

The triumph of antibiotics over many infectious diseases exemplifies the metaphor with which most physicians are comfortable: disease as enemy, the physician as soldier. Their training has taught them to regard any deviation from objective science about the same way as the religious regard sin. The model of disease as an alien invader keeps them from accepting illness, the complaints, as anywhere near real. Yet to understand how placebos work, we must think of disease as the interaction between organic processes and a patient's response. Reaction to a disease may be as crucial as the disease itself.

Illness, then, is a patient's complaint, regardless of whether the origin is biologically detectable. Illness may or may not originate in a disease, but it is the subjective component. Disease may be silent, without symptoms, but it stands for the quantifiable, biologically visible aspects. Disorder—as in *eating disorder*—strikes a useful minor chord, somewhere between the poles. This distinction is crucial to evaluating what placebos do, for illness is all that placebos help.

When pain is treated as a disease on its own, the distinction between disease and illness blurs. If pain goes away, many conclude that a disease has been helped, although it may be only foreboding or annoyance or tribulation that has been lessened.

The Doctor's Casebook
The Irritable Bowel

Many healthy people have diarrhea or constipation with accompanying abdominal pain for much of their lives, especially at times of stress. Many accept disordered bowel function as normal (which I think it is) and do not go to a doctor, whereas a few search incessantly for medical help. Anxiety must have something to do with the choice: in one study people who went to the doctor about abdominal pain were more likely to ascribe it to stress than were others with similar complaints who did not seek out doctors. Why they finally decided to seek help is, of course, a question that compels recognition of the parental role of physicians.

Most physicians can recognize an irritable bowel, particularly in a young person, just by listening. They very likely will not rest with that, however, for they have learned to carry out diagnostic studies to prove the diagnosis. The irritable bowel identified by symptoms alone remains too vague for some physicians until labeled by special wave patterns that can be scrutinized on strips of paper and passed from hand to hand. Indeed, it is now labeled a disease, irritable bowel *disease*, a promotion that makes it more than a reaction to the stresses of life. Over the past few decades the number of diseases that are recognized by symptoms, by what the patient says, have shrunk as training emphasizes the precision of technology. Doctors now hope that the findings of neurobiology will enable them to cast all functional diseases into a morphological mold by finding an abnormality in brain or gene responsible.

Peptic Ulcer

Discussions of peptic ulcer focus on the dose and frequency of antibiotics or acid-suppressing agents and on the harm from aspirin, smoking, and alcohol. No longer is there any interest in the emotional life of patients. Only older physicians still nod in agreement when asked whether stress is important in the recurrences of peptic ulcer. Such issues are ignored partly because physicians think they can do so little about them. Emotions are hard to measure, but the ulcer crater is easy to inspect. Doctors talk to a patient with peptic ulcer very little differently from the way William Osler and other nineteenth-century predecessors might have, but if they rely only on Osler's hundred-year-old treatments, the lawyers would soon be at the door. Psychiatry may have given new visions of why a man or woman gets an ulcer, but science has brought therapy so effective that doctors no longer need to listen to the patients, who understand much less about themselves as a result.

Ulcerative Colitis

Years ago, recovery from ulcerative colitis came about slowly and with much effort by physician and patient to understand the illness; no one was quite certain whether remission was the result of its natural history or came from the patient-physician relationship. Once steroids speeded up the healing process, the work of the physician became very much easier; three to five days of intravenous medication brought about a remission that before might have taken months. People with the disease now get better much more quickly than before, but they know much less about themselves than they used to, and their doctors are glad to be rid of the burden of exploring causes in the mind and life of the patient. Such examples strengthen the idea that the patient's notion of what is wrong can be ignored (and the doctor's too, for that matter) once an injection or a pill eliminates the problem.

Brain or Mind

In the past the body was seen as a machine, and the mind, in Arthur Koestler's adaptation of Plato, as "the ghost in the machine." Now the brain is seen as a computer running the body machine. Physicians find little place for wonder or ecstasy, only reason and objectivity. Training makes them happy to accept the idea that brain-events are mind-events. When they read that calcium flux and changes in an enzyme called cyclic AMP account for memory in the mollusk, they expect that ultimately all human behavior will be reduced to molecular events. Mental illness is no longer the product of malign social forces but "biologically based brain disease."

Physicians do not ask the locus of hope or fear, or free will, but expect that all emotions will someday be reduced to a search in the computer of the brain. They applaud the idea that even grammar is innate, a specialized traceable hardware that will eventually be made visible. They would agree that "there is no disease without a seat, [or] . . . functions without organs." They would disagree with the philosopher Stanley Cavell, who said, "We don't know whether the mind is best represented by the phenomenon of pain, or by that of envy, or by working on a jigsaw puzzle, or by a ringing in the ears."

Scientists confidently expect that someday the human brain will be mapped, each neuron traced to its connections, the computer network laid out to show the places of hope and love, of all our aspirations, that passion will turn out to be a neurotransmitted program. Depression offers a good current example: once deemed the result of repressed anger, now it seems to be an error in the serotonin re-uptake system, to be relieved by chemicals.[3] What is true of depression, they claim, will someday also be true of sorrow, or heroism, for that matter. Investigators have displayed the detailed anatomy and connections of the 302 neurons that make up the brain of a one-millimeter worm, C. elegans. Those 302 neurons, divided into 118 types, make 8,000 connections throughout the worm's body. Laying all this out is the first step, the reductionists hope, toward understanding the human mind.

Physicians and scientists have begun to trace out shifting mechanisms hard-wired like a computer; emotions are different programs that switch functioning circuits. That metaphor would have been unlikely before computers, but newer discoveries may lead to newer models of the brain that resemble what happens when a flock of birds swirl together or a school of fish swim by, turning as one. Perhaps the brain will prove to be more like a school of fish than a computer, and intuition will find its analogue in the sudden eddying of birds rather than the lighting up of circuits.

Even when we understand the brain's circuitry, we will still need the words of a poet. W. H. Auden was no reductionist when he wrote:

> If all a top physicist knows
> About the Truth be true
>
> .   .   .
>
> We have a better time
> Then the Greater Nebulae do,
> Or the atoms in our brains

The mind-brain split is bewildering. How easy it would be if thought were secreted by the brain like insulin from the pancreas. Is the brain a pancreas or a computer? Dreams can be traced to specific neuronal activity, suggesting that brain structures produce psychological function and behavior. The human brain is so much bigger and so much more complicated than the little worm's. So-called cortical columns run up and down parts of the human brain for a very short way; there are at least 600 million columns, each containing about 110 neurons, 50 billion neurons in that tiny area alone. Beyond my comprehension lie the brain circuits that may "generate emotion, link emotion to perception, and provide an impetus to behavior." Magnetic resonance imaging and positron-emission tomography studies of the brain with radioactive tracer molecules promise "a new set of eyes" to examine the chemistry of the mind. Will we find charity there?

Such anatomic determinism finds all human emotions in models of the brain or faults of the gene. But a single gene, altered or absent, is not the same as a disease, which requires far more than one defect; thousands of genes make up a genome, so that usually when one goes awry, others compensate. One gene is hardly responsible for poverty or depression, a fact that makes Stephen Rose ask for a more "integrated understanding of the relationships between the biological, personal and social." Diseases are both biological and social in origin: even though alcoholism and obesity may find their origin in our genes, their control lies within the compass of our will. We are not always prisoners of our parents and their genes, unless we inherit a neuromuscular catastrophe like Lou Gehrig's disease.

How the mind emerges from the brain is beyond me, and where the spirit finds its home I do not know. I continue to think mind and brain are as different as illness and disease and am a little fearful of future discoveries.

The Patient as a Whole

In the Middle Ages, doctors tried to repair the body and left the mind, behavior, religion, and the soul to the church, just as modern scientific reductionists ignore the psychic and psychosocial extensions of disease. Thoughtful postmodern physicians, often trained as psychiatrists, have long promoted the idea of the patient as a person without wide success, even when recast by George Engel as the biopsychosocial medical model, or systems medicine. In this model, body and mind influence each other, and an ulcer is more than a break in the stomach lining—it is a breakdown in a person with specific social, emotional, and economic stresses. Modern gastroenterologists have paid little attention to such holistic and contextual matters, finding their justification in using antibiotics to eliminate peptic ulcer.

Hard Versus Soft Science

Doctors can do little about social systems. Surveying the social cataclysms of the twentieth century, they fear that social sciences have made little difference to our world; in medical science, in contrast, they find the reassurance of hard science and delight in how vastly science and technology have improved their knowledge and practice. Doctors know little more today about why an alcoholic drinks than they did fifty years ago, but now they can plumb the pancreas with a scope to lay out its ducts and use computed tomography to outline its contour. Physicians pore over their scientific journals for explanations of disease and how to treat it, but put aside as too soft anything that has to do with people and society. Physicians are pragmatists who look for information to cure patients but who have little patience and less time to understand those patients.

In daily practice physicians come gradually to recognize the importance of sociocultural and economic factors, which they have not been trained to deal with. Like lawyers fresh out of law school who have studied the Constitution and legal theory but are ill equipped to accept the reality of plea bargaining, medical students learn the care of acute disease, but the person remains a phantom until people begin to turn up in the office or clinic. And these people are far more complicated to deal with than disease. "Any attempt to understand why the patient feels and acts in a particular manner must include an inquiry into his subjective interpretation of what is happening to him—and to his personal meaning of events related to his illness. . . . In general, the more the meaning of disease and its symptoms is influenced by unconscious factors, the more irrational, idiosyncratic, and unpredictable is the patient's overt response likely to be" (Lipowski 1969).

Humanity and Humanities in Medicine

Common sense is needed for a social model of disease. That is why novelists and writers are important for physicians; they illustrate how it feels to be sick and portray the inner life of patients. Writers explore that other world where the poet explains death and life better than the physicist. The novelist gives medical readers distance to reflect on life and death without having to act on what they think.

To interpret the light and shadow of an X-ray or CAT scan requires training, experience, and knowledge of more than what is displayed. To understand a poem requires more than seeing it on paper. The more poetry one has read, the richer the responses, and the deeper the meanings derived. To read a poem requires as much experience as to read an MRI. To understand a patient, a physician need not have read Henry James or Dostoyevsky, but physicians who have read widely are more likely to be aware of tones and shades, the nuances that a less well read physician might pass by. Like aging, reading brings experience.

The Metaphors of Disease

The prevailing metaphor of medicine—doctor as scientist or soldier —leads to the concept of disease as a physical object, especially an alien invader. The movie *Invasion of the Body Snatchers* caught the tone: People become alien to themselves as aliens convert human bodies, outwardly unchanged, to their own uses. The seed pods of alien invaders are the source of disease, just like H. pylori. What the patient says is unreliable because that person has been contaminated.

Patients feel what is going on inside themselves, but they cannot always find the words to tell others. Their symptoms are interpreted by a physician immersed in a medical culture in which the eye is more important than the ear. Metaphors like the "mind's eye" and the "eye of faith" remind us of the long reliance on seeing in Western culture.

Following Wittgenstein, Arthur Kleinman contrasts the "straight regular streets" of scientific language with the twisting streets of ordinary language: "Our language can be seen as an ancient city: a maze of little streets and squares, of old and new houses, and of houses with additions from various periods; and this surrounded by a multitude of new boroughs with straight regular streets and uniform houses." Medical theorists pay major attention to the "wide, well-designed and clearly mapped suburban avenues" of biophysical science, embarrassed at the "archaic route of medicine, which strikes us as most like the twisting, narrow, unmapped streets and clutter of old and new houses of the ancient inner city." Psychiatrists still listen to what patients have to say, for they know that talking strengthens empathy, but they are as besieged by case managers as the Bishop of Bingen in his mouse-tower on the Rhine.

Diagnosis: The Eye and the Ear

Patients want to tell the doctor about their illness, but some doctors and some patents find such conversation too personal. Asked to imagine being a patient, college students had no objection to their bodies being probed or even photographed, but having their words recorded or taped seemed an intrusion: "That's too private," one complained. "I don't need to let my doctor know what I am thinking."

Thoughts reflected in conversation are important to understanding illness. Talk is intimate; the tongue has a direct connection with the thoughts, closer than the spleen's. If I tell you what I am thinking or what I fear, you know me, more than if you biopsy my liver, hold my heart in your hands, or even read my EEG.

Seeing and Talking

Physicians talk a lot with each other about cancer and what to do about it and much less with the patients who have it. That is left to social workers,psychiatrists, and nurses. At gastrointestinal conferences at Yale, pathologists and radiologists are always in attendance to teach us gastroenterologists about image and structure; but social workers are not there, and psychiatrists are almost never invited. My colleagues want hard facts and visual images. They want to learn all they can about technological ways to help their patients, not discuss illness, and those in training quickly learn to ask for images instead of asking questions of patients. Fortunately, more and more postmodern physicians doubt that all diseases will be explained by a switch turned on or off by some gene.

Physicians love to show each other printouts or pictures of what they have seen. Those little icons of disease, those X-rays and echoes and scans, give a picture to the pains of the patient, but one that has been safely sterilized. The image carries none of the anguish of some-one telling us of pain. It is easier to look at films in an X-ray department far from the patient than to listen to someone complaining, for when the patient is through, the doctor has only the memory of what has been said. After the patient has been to the X-ray or endoscopic depart-ment, there is a picture to look at over and over.

Concepts of disease change when imaging techniques show the disease. A patient's complaints are evanescent, at least to the physician; they are words uttered, listened to, which quickly "float away on the air," in Walter Ong's lovely phrase. X-rays, sonograms, endoscopic photographs, even numbers from a laboratory, are far more perma-nent. They fix the disease, give it a reality, make physicians think of it as a thing that can be named.

Physicians have always delighted in giving names to complaints, even in ancient times. In the *Republic*, book III, Plato comments: "By indolence and a habit of life such as we have been describing, men fill themselves with waters and winds, as if their bodies were a marsh, compelling the ingenious sons of Asclepius to find more names for diseases, such as flatulence and catarrh; is not this, too, a disgrace? 'Yes,' he said, 'they do certainly give very strange and newfangled names to diseases.' "

A long time ago a neurologist warned, "It is often better not to gratify the craving for nomenclature that is manifested by many patients, but rather to explain to them that to give ailments a definite name would involve more error than truth" (Gowers). As Thomas Szasz has put it, "Diagnoses are not diseases." The label of a diagnosis does not create a disease even if it pleases doctor and patient. What one generation named soldier's heart, another called neurocirculatory asthenia; today we say posttraumatic stress syndrome. Just as the diagnosis of hysteria vanished partly because doctors decided to give the collection of complaints a different name, so physicians and laypeople alike must be wary of searching too hard for a specific diagnosis. A name does not bring health with it. Nor should relief by an antidepressant be taken to imply that a disease is present. That the premenstrual syndrome can be alleviated by Prozac does not mean that premenstrual syndrome is a brain disease.

To many physicians, an ulcer displayed on an endoscopic photo is something to act on with assurance, far more than if they just deduce it from the patient's story. Suggest that they treat ulcer dyspepsia for ten days, postponing diagnostic tests and investigating only patients who do not improve, and academicians will complain that medicine is a science and will warn that they must know what they are treating. They feel uncomfortable inferring from a patient's complaint and not proving what is present by seeing it.

Managed care companies are also after visual proof of what they pay for. To confirm to their lay overseers what their ears have already heard, physicians may need to do more procedures rather than fewer. That is no real change, because when they were paid for piecework, physicians used to shoot for the highest-paid diagnosis.

Seeing the Disease

The imaging explosion allows the display of normal anatomy and disease in an ever more detailed way. When physicians think of a disease only in terms of its anatomical expression, they risk reifying it —thinking of it only as a thing. When that happens, the primacy of anatomy is once again asserted, as it was when anatomists first dissected out and named what they found in cadavers.

Before X-rays provided the first major imaging revolution that opened up the body, surgeons had to draw pictures of what they found. Speculums had helped them look into vagina, rectum, and throat; with newer instruments they scrutinized eyes and ears. X-rays were easy to understand—the bones looked just like a skeleton—and yet the black and white plates showed the living body in ways never before imagined. An X-ray quickly provided a more authoritative diagnosis than just listening to the patient. X-ray techniques strengthened the notion of the body as a machine, as Joel Howell has pointed out. I remember the little porcelain statues on which modest Chinese women would point out to a physician where they hurt. X-rays provided a new way, devoid of sexual embarrassment, to locate those pains.

Looking at X-ray pictures on scan or film is quicker and easier than deducing the problem from the patient's complaints. That in turn strengthens the conviction that understanding comes mainly from improved techniques rather than from reflection or conversation. Reading a story is different from hearing it from an old man talking to a grandchild; the change is from intuition and magic to science and reason.

Such technical advances need not lead to silence between patient and physician. Instead of advising the patient that there is probably nothing wrong but ordering some tests just to be sure, many physicians order the tests without explanation. After organs and tissues and fluids test normal, they order more, until the patient begins to fear that something hidden will finally be uncovered by the right test.

If the first evaluation does not suggest something dire, it is unlikely that anything serious will turn up in even a long follow-up. That is not always true, but those rare events provide little excuse for routinely testing everything. That is where placebos may be useful and where the serotonin receptor re-uptake inhibitors, such as the tricyclic antidepressives, have been so helpful in relieving pain and making further testing unnecessary.

Visceral Sensitivity

Up against complaints for which they can find no valid physiological explanations, physicians have begun to recognize that some people are more sensitive to the inner workings of their body than others. I give great credit to artists, actors, poets, and other imaginative people who in their work have to be sensitive to life. It is not surprising that they should be more sensitive to bodily functions as well. Such heightened awareness is now denominated the visceral pain syndrome, of which the "sensitive heart" is one of the latest examples. Cardiologists have been particularly eager to find a site in the body for every pain; when people complain of chest pain without evidence of anatomic abnormality, these specialists talk of heightened visceral pain sensitivity but do the angiograms anyway.

One of the very important contributions of complementary medicine is the responsibility given to patients to do something for themselves, even if it is no more than deciding to ignore an ache or pain when the doctor finds nothing wrong. Placebos help some people to strengthen that healthy resolve.

Acute Cholecystitis

Clinicians who recognize acute cholecystitis by its characteristics are dumbfounded to learn that clinical features are less reliable than ultrasound and radio-nuclide study. It may be that physicians should rely only on images, but reliance may reflect inexperience. If doctors are taught to recognize acute appendicitis only by computed tomography (CT) scan, that will influence the way the disorder is detected and thought about. Ordering such scans and studies in anyone with a pain between knee and chest to rule out an unlikely possibility is lazy clinical diagnosis. By using accurate imaging techniques this way, the concept of acute cholecystitis or acute appendicitis as clinically detectable diseases fades; worse, the idea that a clinician can learn anything useful from talking to the patient seems ever more ludicrous.

Categories

Classifications and models tell us something about the concerns of a society. In a wet country, rain is particularized as *shower, mist, downpour, sprinkle*—terms that are meaningless to desert nomads. Cynthia Ozick describes the scorn of the eastern European Jew for the Christian categorization of knives: "By them they got sword, they got lance, they got halberd . . . cutlass, pike, rapier, foil, ten dozen more."

In considering diagnostic errors, Western physicians have room for only two categories, based on the presence or absence of detectable disease. There is no category for visualizing a problem that doesn't really matter to the patient, such as a cyst in the liver, or for overemphasizing the importance of cholesterol levels in the elderly. There is too much reliance on visible abnormalities, with too little concern for their significance.

Observer Variation

Observer variation sets important limits to medical vision: even when people look at the same object, they will differ about what they see or say. Presumably few would disagree about a circle, but in one study, ten pathologists disagreed about a series of slides 20 to 30 percent of the time. Identifying the reasons for error in seeing and describing something has become a science of its own, even for a sense as transparently accurate as the eye.

Listening to Patients

Speaking is the consciousness of another person. Sound penetrates, but because it so quickly dissipates, we have to keep listening, not just hear. Sight and its frozen counterpart, the image, are more permanent. We can look at images again and again. It is easier to bring the picture back to the mind's eye than to its ear. Few physicians (besides psychiatrists) have ever deemed a patient's words important enough to capture on tape—maybe, as college students have reminded me, because it would be a violation of their privacy in a way that liver scans are not.

We hear the real person when we listen. Listening brings immediacy, at least face-to-face. A voice over the telephone or an audiotape is somehow different: I must concentrate more when I do not see the face. The way doctors ask questions is as important as what the patient tells them. The story changes a little each time it is told, and it is told differently to different doctors. For some physicians, such variations make the story soft data, not as reliable as the hard copy of the image.

But I find that very repetition of the story helpful when I am puzzled, especially when someone is not responding to therapy. The second account is often not the same as the first, and the new elements give new clues. Moreover, empathy and empathic listening help healing, and so they come in for increasing praise from postmodern doctors. Just as surgeons increase their ability with experience, so listening —whether reflecting what is heard or free-floating—improves with practice. Some people are better at listening than others, probably out of natural empathy, but giving patients time to talk helps to release emotions that, confined, exacerbate complaints.

Emotion

Medical images freeze the idea of disease, and, worse, they sterilize disease. They bring the objectivity that physicians prize, but they make disease abstract. Not only have doctors lost the complaints of the sick, but they have lost senses beyond sight: smell, touch, hearing. Wordsworth called poetry emotion "recollected in tranquillity," and disease is as trapped on film as emotions are in poetry (although poetry can also release emotions). Images make suffering more endurable for the physician. Once the radiologist had to touch patients to X-ray them, but now computed tomography and magnetic resonance imaging, the new developments of telemedicine, make it possible for images of the patient's body to be reconstructed through the air of cyberspace, with the radiologist a thousand miles away in an imaging department. Physicians often turn to radiologists for answers more as supplicants than as colleagues. No one puts the patient back together after the complaints have been fractured into MRI, US, CT, IDA, and all the rest of the alphabetical tests. The postmodern generation is said to be different; doctors reared amid the jumble of cyberspace may turn out to be better than their older modern colleagues at putting patients back together holistically.

Physician as Mediator

The physician must act as interpreter of a patient's complaint, mediator between human and machine, between complaint and image. To do this, the physician must first listen to what the patient has to say. There are blind physicians, but I have never run into one deaf from birth. A deaf person might become a splendid radiologist or surgeon but cannot break through that communication barrier that many may feel when someone cannot hear what they want to tell. To test the truth of this, try reading poetry to someone hard-of-hearing. The voice tells so much. Physicians hypnotized by images should look on images as freeing them from the constraints of the physical examination, giving them more time to listen, to talk with their patients. Instead, they see more patients or order more studies. Sadly, however, when I tell these things to gastrointestinal trainees, they smile, for they have been taught that the images are all that count.

The image is not the patient. Marshall McLuhan puts it vividly. "Suppose that, instead of displaying the Stars and Stripes, we were to write the words 'American flag' across a piece of cloth and to display that. While the symbols would convey the same meaning, the effect would be quite different."

Grand Rounds

Grand Rounds exemplify the changes in medicine. They began as a tour around the wards by the chief physician and his associates, with each patient the center of the discussion. Grand Rounds moved to an amphitheater when too many physicians began to attend. Patients were brought to the conference so that physicians could have someone to talk to and see. The discussion was personal, oral, informed, and patient-centered.

Gradually the aim of Grand Rounds shifted; not problem patients but interesting cases were discussed. The particular patient became less important than the disease, and growing concern for patients' rights and privacy made displaying sick people at a conference seem a breach of privacy. Less and less time was given to the patients, until they became icons of themselves, present like the American flag. Anyone could have represented the patient, for all the good it did to bring patients to Grand Rounds.

From the case it is not far to statistics, organs, and the apparatus of reductionism. Grand Rounds in most hospitals have become lectures with only rarely the pretense of a patient's story. The speaker points to slides projected on a screen, reading from them as from any paper. Yet the logic of a written paper is quite different from the logic of a talk to an audience. A Grand Rounds audience is supposed to listen. Printed handouts are distributed for later review. Physicians rely on the written word almost as much as on the image and have only to see something in print to believe it.

The Religion of Vision

William Meyer emphasizes the American "religion of vision": "The English ear has been killed by the American eye, the divine work has been usurped by the divine vision." The eagle with its eagle eye, the mystic eye of the seal emblazoned on the dollar bill, the Statue of Liberty with its lamp—all tell us how everything in the United States is interpreted by the eye. The same theme runs from the early poets, whose religious experiences were often visual, to Ralph Waldo Emerson, who called the American a "transparent eyeball." The word, the mysteries of the unseen, have been bleached out in modern America by the light of the television set, but it may be returning with the printed dialogue of e-mail.

The reliance on vision is not strictly American. The entire scientific approach depends on what Ong has called hypervisualism—the notion that all sensations can be reduced to vision through such devices as charts and measurements. The image isolates the patient from the physician, just as sight isolates and freeze-frames, whereas sound penetrates and pours into the listener. Scientific medicine isolates the patient from the physician and lets the physician remain silent. Physicians feel triumph at seeing on X-ray film what they had predicted, for the mystery is solved, the problem visualized. Listening to the story unfold, learning from the patient the cause of pain, does not give most physicians the same thrill. The Greeks somewhere said that the eye was for accuracy, but the ear was for truth.[4] To understand a sight requires organized preconception, but listening demands thoughtful synthesis of what the patient tells.

What Care Means

Most physicians look for disease rather than listen to patients. Yet illness can be understood best by listening to what is being said. Drugs help disease, but words can help illness. No one can see an illness.

Modern physicians do not listen to the difference between "I *see* what you say" and "I *hear* what you say," as Ong has suggested. Students learn about diseases by reading references and textbooks, although they could learn almost as much by watching caring physicians while serving in something between an apprenticeship, in which they do, and a discipleship, in which they learn to say. Images can free physicians from the constraints of the physical examination and give them more time to listen to the patient. Listening is much harder work than seeing; it takes time, concentration, and active participation. But physicians need to listen as much as to look, to make all senses work together.

Stephen Schmidt, a professor of pastoral studies at Loyola University in Chicago, has written about his own Crohn's disease in a poem that reveals what care really means.

When You Come into My Room (abridged)

When you come into my hospital room, you need to know that I love earthy sensuous life, beauty, travel, eating, drinking, J&B scotch

. . . loving, the wonder and awe of sexual intimacy . . . that I have Crohn's disease and 3 small-bowel resections . . . that I am chronically ill, and am seeking healing, not cure . . . that I can travel only where there is modern technology . . . that I hate rounds held outside my room, rounds that do not include nurses, my wife, my children, my pastor, or even me . . . rounds done over me, around me, but not with me . . . that I am anxious about aging and how I will cope, that I long for one perfect day, only one symptom-free 24 hours, that I lust for remission . . . that I seek meaning in suffering . . . that I have faith and lose it . . . that I am slowly coming to believe that meaning is what we bring to suffering, not what we gain from it, that God, faith, meaning, ultimate concern, love, salvation are the being of my being, that I struggle with God. . . . When you come into my room, . . . you need to know all this if you want to heal me and bear my rage about my disease that I will never be cured, that my daughter has Crohn's disease and is only 33 years old, that she too has had her first surgery. . . . When you come into my hospital room . . . keep hope alive, it is all I have.

The placebo response and the placebo effect provide the climax of our drama, in two scenes, one called illness and the other, disease. The scenes distinguish the response of the patient to the placebo from its effect on disease, if any. What the patient feels after a placebo is different from remission of disease.

The placebo effect has been defined as "any effect attributable to a pill, potion, or procedure, but not to its pharmacodynamic or specific properties." Because one can never be sure what all those properties are, Howard Brody has defined it further as "the change in the patient's condition that is attributable to the symbolic import of the healing intervention rather than to the intervention's specific pharmacologic or physiologic effects." This describes what I am calling the placebo response. The definition makes the person's response count for more than the response of the disease. The placebo response is the mind change in the person receiving the medication—little different, I expect, from that in the person receiving complementary medical help. Because placebos affect illness, not disease, it is helpful to distinguish response from effect. Most minor diseases get better on their own, so a patient who takes a pill or potion when he or she feels the worst will give the pill credit for natural improvement. Even cancer may, very rarely, undergo spontaneous remission, which means that more than a single anecdote is needed to convince me that a response is predictable, not just a coincidence.

chapter six

What

Placebos

Can Do

Claims About Placebos

Preexisting Symptoms

Before ideas about informed consent precluded some psychological experiments, investigators often noted that the side effects of placebos in controlled trials resembled those of the active drug. Two explanations were obvious: (1) these side effects were found because that is what investigators were looking for, or (2) they represented preexisting complaints.

To test these explanations, in the 1960s some investigators told experimental subjects that they were determining the side effects of a new drug, but did not tell them that they were taking placebos nor what the expected side effects might be. Gastrointestinal complaints loomed large beforehand: heartburn, nausea, and abdominal pain were not infrequent; dizziness, blurred vision, dry mouth, palpitation, urinary frequency, and drowsiness were also reported. After taking the placebos, the subjects complained that their previous gastrointestinal symptoms had increased in frequency and severity. "The only new symptom elicited by placebos was vomiting." Drowsiness, dizziness, and other complaints also increased with the number of pills taken.[1]

Patients in a retirement center grew so alarmed about their symptoms that their nurses asked that the drugs be stopped because of their toxic effects. This very illuminating study concluded: "The ability of placebos to intensify the apparent severity of such pre-treatment symptoms and to elicit them in others in whom they had not pre-existed, suggest that the active administrating of medication may so focus the subject's attention introspectively that some complaints previously given little or no attention are magnified to a degree where they become regarded as 'side effects' of the medication being given."

In many other clinical trials the placebo response has been influenced by the severity of the initial complaints, in part because physicians, like others, find what they are looking for: placebos that are being compared to stimulants will increase energy and even heart rate, whereas placebos tested against sedatives will do just the opposite. All this happens as a result of the suggestibility of the patient, another example of the strong influence of expectation. This notion has been supported by a concluding analysis from the University of Connecticut: what depressed people expect from an antidepressant like Prozac plays a dominant role in ensuring a favorable response, twice as strong as the pharmacological effect itself.

Cancer Studies

One of the most dramatic reports of remissions by a placebo, many times referred to, even today, is much less impressive on review.[2] A psychologist, Bruno Klopfer, first told the story more than forty years ago in a presidential address to the Society for Projective Techniques. He had not seen the patient, but quoted the account by a Dr. Philip West, otherwise unidentified.

A patient of unknown age, Mr. Wright had a generalized "far-advanced malignancy involving the lymph nodes, lymphosarcoma. . . .Huge tumor masses, the size of oranges, were in the neck, axillas, groins, chest and abdomen." The patient was given a course of Krebiozen, a purported cancer cure of the 1950s, with great enthusiasm. After one injection, the physician wrote, "What a surprise was in store for me! I had left him febrile, gasping for air, completely bedridden. Now, here he was, walking around the ward chatting happily with the nurses. . . . The tumor masses had melted like snowballs on a hot stove and in only these few days, they were half their original size!"

Reports, however, began to appear that Krebiozen was of no value: "This disturbed our Mr. Wright considerably as the weeks wore on. . . . He began to lose faith in his last hope which so far had been life-saving and left nothing to be desired. As the reported results became increasingly dismal, his faith waned and after two months of practically perfect health, he relapsed to his original state, and became very gloomy and miserable."

At this point the physician "decided to take the chance and play the quack. So deliberately lying, I told him not to believe what he read in the papers, the drug was really most promising after all. . . . I administered the first injection of the doubly potent, fresh preparation—consisting of fresh water and nothing more. The results of this experiment were quite unbelievable to us at the time. . . . Tumor masses melted, chest fluid vanished, he became ambulatory.'' The water injections were continued, since they had worked such wonders and the patient remained symptom-free over two months. Then, "the final AMA announcement appeared in the press—Nationwide tests show Krebiozen to be a worthless drug in the treatment of cancer. . . . Within a few days of this report, Mr. Wright was readmitted to the hospital in extremis . . . and he succumbed in less than two days" (Klopfer).

Obviously there were no objective data beyond the secondhand testimonial. Not only was the physician unknown, but only the story was presented, which makes it easy to conjecture that much of the drama was enthusiastic interpretation. The patient felt better, but without better documentation we should not perpetuate the notion that placebos can dissolve the objective manifestations of cancer, any more than we accept many other testimonials without data.

In another case, reported in the general cheer of Christmas Day some years ago in my hometown paper, the *New Haven Register*, a woman apparently lived for two years after being diagnosed with pancreatic cancer, much longer than had been expected, thanks to visualization techniques. It turned out that the diagnosis was made not by biopsies but by palpation, a technique no more accurate than tossing a coin. The patient was grateful, but I remain skeptical.

Sometimes, for reasons no one understands, the growth of some cancers slows, and a very few even disappear.[3] Those occurrences are so rare as to raise doubts about most reported spontaneous cures of cancer. A remarkable review a long time ago from the University of Illinois brought together 176 reports of proven cancers that had disappeared or at least grown smaller. Spontaneous regression was defined as "partial or complete disappearance of malignant tumor in the absence of all treatment" or after treatment inadequate to account for the cure. More than half the remissions involved cancers of the kidney, the nervous system, skin (malignant melanoma), and the uterus and ovaries. Unfortunately, no one stated how long the spontaneous regression had lasted or whether it was permanent; reports were usually published shortly after the improvement had been noted, a testimony to the enthusiasm of doctors for the miraculous.

Reports of spontaneous regression warn of how much caution is needed in accepting the efficacy of any therapeutic measure that purports to cure cancer. Some cancers disappear for uncertain reasons, but consistency and predictability are key. Consistency is lacking in most claims of cures by faith healing or alternative forms of therapy, or even by more mainline therapies. Some cancers do shrink, some do regress, but consistency must be demanded from the proponents of any cure.

Laypeople and some physicians do not realize how difficult it sometimes is for pathologists to agree on the presence of a cancer. Unfortunately, cancer cells can be mistaken for rapidly growing but otherwise normal cells engaged in repair. That must account for a lot of the disagreement about the results of therapy. Whenever a miracle cure is said to have occurred, several observers need to review the material.

The Mind-Body Connection

For a long time now, physicians and psychologists have tried to confirm the mind-body hypothesis for disease by proving that persons can will their way to health, or at the very least can stimulate their immune system through thinking. After all, the very explicit reasoning runs, if the pituitary gland is embedded in the brain and if it monitors and controls so many hormones and neurological connections, it should be able to marshal armies of immune cells to deal with cancer. I compare the pathological forces of cancer to the Nazi armies that ravaged Europe: they overwhelmed small countries from Norway to Greece in no time at all. Whatever influence the mind has over the immune system in health is likely to be as ineffective as the Dutch trying to repel the Germans.[4]

Still, people want to know that they are in charge of their destiny; the medical literature reveals a persistent optimism in regard to cancer, a pervasive unreality that goes back many years. David Spiegel and colleagues in California have shown that women with breast cancer who maintained a fighting spirit or an optimistic outlook lived longer than those who were depressed. Their evidence, that psychological help improves the outlook, received much acclaim and received enormous foundation support, partly, a skeptic supposes, because foundations need publicity to show that their grants are well spent and partly because reassurance is what everyone likes to read about and believe. We are all looking for medical miracles and, of course, there have been many in this century. Yet headlines shout about preliminary successes but ignore the failures that often follow. Whereas in the nineteenth century the religious went to search for cures at shrines, in the twentieth, patients go to doctors and psychologists; they hunt for the same satisfactions in California as once they did in Quebec at the shrine of Ste. Anne de Beaupré.

We all need purposes and groups, and gain support from finding and talking with others like us in the same spot. The Spiegel group of researchers are optimistic about their research, and women—all of us, really—want to believe them. When studies like the one reported in the *Journal of the National Cancer Institute* in 1996 come along to show no obvious relation between depression or any other psychological state and the survival of women with breast cancer, the authors offer the usual confession that maybe they did not do their studies right or that subtle changes might not have been detected. That ritual caution feeds the public's hope, the way the doctor does who tells a patient that "there is always hope" in order to keep the patient's spirits up. Any very subtle changes that require sophisticated psychological and statistical methods to detect will mean very little to survival. The soldiers of the Dutch army may have been more agile than the hordes of Nazis, but they were overwhelmed by sheer numbers. Nevertheless, given the inherent optimism of us all, pilgrimages for miracles of the mind will continue, and skepticism will arouse only annoyance.

In health, the mind-body connection is real, and it can right an illness and does. Although we can talk ourselves into love or even charity, we cannot slow down a cancer by will or hope alone. Placebos may help symptoms, but they do not help diseases. What mattered for the breast cancer patients was the number of lymph nodes involved and their estrogen receptor status. The investigators recognized, however, that adherence to a therapeutic regimen also counted. Those who followed a regimen the best were generally those with fighting spirit who searched for ways to procure the best therapy. Women who were fighters did what they were told to do by the doctors. Doing what the doctor tells you is likely to help more than not. The chemotherapeutic program is more important than healthy thoughts.

The journalist Bill Moyers had a discussion about cancer with Michael Lerner, founder and president of the Commonweal Cancer Help Program in California, who has devoted considerable thought and study to the problem. Moyers said, "The parallel assumption would be that the healing process you focus on here would help the body dispose of cancer." The healing process covered all so-called healing interventions. Lerner sensibly resisted agreement. "It's very difficult in any circumstances to completely reverse that. Mainstream medicine does not have cures for metastatic cancer. So we should start with the fact that if we look at all the people using all the different alternative healing methods with cancer, we find relatively few well-documented cases where people have fully reversed a cancer, and it has never returned."

Physiological Effects of Placebos

Most observers accept the idea that placebos can lead to impressive physiological changes, from lowering blood pressure to reducing high blood-sugar levels. The nature of the evidence and the time frame of many of these observations, especially early reports of placebo response in the laboratory, can be regarded with some skepticism.

Many studies were carried out in the 1940s on Tom, a man with a permanent opening on his belly wall into his stomach, which made its contents easy to study. Abdominal discomfort and reddening of his stomach folds followed his ingestion of "three large imposing-looking red capsules." Tom was under considerable stress: "Following ingestion of certain of the substances which seemed to induce special anxiety, he often noted abdominal cramps and diarrhea which could not be attributed to the effect of the drug. This disturbance began following an experiment in which he ingested 0.015 gm prostigmine. The cramps and diarrhea in this instance were doubtless due to the pharmacological action of the drug." The red capsules, however, contained "only starch and lactose." After Tom had swallowed them, he "noted mild abdominal cramps and an urgent need to defecate. . . . He promptly had one loose stool and his face continued to be red for half an hour. He expressed extreme anxiety regarding the content of the capsules and at this time he was reassured that they contained only milk sugar."

Half a century later, when doctors know that lactose produces diarrhea in many people, we cannot conclude that the placebo was inactive. The earlier conclusions might have reflected the intuition or the expectation of the observers, as well as the possibility that Tom, working as an assistant in the very laboratory where he was being studied, could not have remained innocent of his employers' expectations. Resentment, more than sterile water, doubled Tom's gastric secretion, for Tom "disliked intensely being pricked by hypodermic needles." Injections of water that the subject hated have little useful to show about placebos; they were important because they did confirm the effect of psychic stimuli on gastric secretion.

The effect of placebos on normal physiology is vastly different from their effect on the pathophysiology of disease. I do not know of any studies of pathophysiological changes in the sick person given placebos as therapy other than as part of a clinical trial.

Emotions influence normal physiological activities; gastric secretion does increase with anger or anxiety. The development of an ulcer, however, reflects forces driving the pathophysiology so hard as to submerge any observable effect of a placebo. Although anger at an injection increased Tom's gastric secretion, evidence that the gastric secretion of duodenal ulcer patients can be similarly affected is far less persuasive. Strong emotions surely affect normal physiology, but we need better evidence that the emotions engendered by placebos have any effect on the pathophysiology that produces disease.

There are many other examples. Ultrasound to relieve the pain and swelling of dental work proved equally effective whether or not the machine was turned on, as long as everyone involved believed that it was emitting sound. A bland placebo ointment relieved pain in other patients, who subsequently became strong placebo responders.

Subject or Patient

Experimental subjects are paid for their time in a laboratory to take pills and report their responses, some pleasant and some unpleasant. An Australian researcher, Michael Jospe, has urged caution: "Such research, and in fact any research on the placebo effect, should not be conducted with nonpatients. Laboratory experiments are not clinical situations. . . . An experimenter is not a therapist, a subject is not a patient, and a laboratory is not a clinic." The intent of investigators is quite different from the intent of clinicians, who are treating real patients.

Placebo responses in a patient with symptoms are quite different from the placebo responses of a subject in a laboratory setting. Receiving pills for a complaint is different from receiving pills that the subject is told may cause an effect—sleepiness, nausea, or a headache. These differences are not always clearly distinguished when all nonphysiological effects are labeled placebo effects and all unpleasant side effects are called nocebos. Many so-called adverse effects of placebos were present before study and were magnified by attention to them during study, as we have already seen.

The patient in chronic pain who has had relief from shots may react quite differently from the patient who has had no relief from placebo shots before. The first of a series of injections often determines how someone will react. People are so different, their history and experiences so personal, that each person represents a unique placebo responder.

Effects on Blood Sugar

It is firmly held that placebos can lower blood sugar levels in diabetics, but even though that may be true, the original study did not permit that flat implication. Doctors treated a group of diabetic patients with an active antidiabetic drug for six months and then repeated the course of treatment. But "after a six month trial, an identical placebo was substituted without acknowledgment to the patient." In the Boston of the 1960s no attempt at informed consent was thought necessary for that substitution.

Many of the patients taking placebos maintained very good long-term control of their diabetes. They came regularly to the clinic and had a close relationship with their physicians, all of which affirms that good care can do much for some diabetics. Nowhere has anyone documented that taking a placebo is followed by a lowered blood sugar level. A placebo might do just that, but the data are not available. Control trials bring astonishingly good relief of pain or healing of duodenal ulcers once the patients come under observation. The benefit of care in any clinical trials must be distinguished from evidence for physiological effects.

Other Disorders

Placebos have been credited with stopping some disease processes largely through psychosomatic connections, suggestion being considered as important as the pills themselves. These data do not, however, withstand modern scrutiny. Placebos reportedly brought relief to many complaints, including coughs, mood changes, angina pectoris, headaches, seasickness, anxiety, hypertension, asthma, depression, and the common cold, all familiar problems resembling those helped by alternative medicine as well. Some papers give traceable references for placebo successes with pain, coughs, mood changes, angina pectoris, and the common cold; there were none for headaches, seasickness, asthma, hypertension, depression, or hyperglycemia. H. R. Bourne made the following cogent point about all diseases in which placebos are said to help: "In these diseases the percentage of patients receiving relief is not so high, but in virtually every study a considerable number of patients are helped by placebo medication. A study that shows no response to placebo might almost be suspected of lack of objectivity on that ground alone."

Overinterpretation

In an influential book, Lying, Sissela Bok implied that pure placebos might kill when she stated: "Worst of all, those children who cannot tolerate antibiotics may have severe reactions, sometimes fatal, to such unnecessary medication." Antibiotics can kill whether or not they are used as placebos; they should not be used as placebos at all. It is not helpful to generalize that death can follow a pure placebo used in the usual fashion when an antibiotic given as a placebo is what killed the patient.

Conclusions are often overstated, as in this example: "Placebo reactions may resemble those of active drugs not only in the end results but also in the patterns of activity. These patterns include a peak effect a certain number of hours after administration of the drug, a cumulative effect of increase in symptom relief as the drug is continued over time, with a carryover effect after the drug is stopped, and a decrease in efficacy as the severity of the symptom increases" (Lasagna). The original study merely reported the effect of aspirin or a placebo on pain relief and the effect of a placebo given to patients with various chronic diseases who were told that the tablets would increase their appetite and improve their pep and energy. Both groups improved with placebo therapy that lasted beyond the time of active-drug administration. Moreover, although the investigators described effects that looked like pharmacological ones, they were studying pain and other subjective phenomena, not more objective events. We should not carry their implications too far.

What Is to Be Measured

To evaluate placebo responses requires deciding what is to be evaluated, whether an objective disease, the lessening of complaints, a change in an organ's shape or size, or a reduction in pain or suffering. I maintain that relief of pain and suffering on a person-to-person level is the important issue. The placebo response may ameliorate diseases, but the evidence is lacking except for subjective reports. That placebos relieve pain is true enough, however, but to look at what kinds of pain are relieved and in what circumstances it is important to classify pain in some reasonable manner (see Chapter 7).

Suffering, anxiety, and much more make up what people call pain. Someone in a dental chair having pain tolerance manipulated by behavioral scientists knows that the pain will be short-lived and is worth enduring, for whatever was wrong will be repaired; in contrast, the patient with a chronic headache may worry about a brain tumor. The experimental subject with arm pain from a heat lamp in the laboratory may have doubts about having volunteered for the study, whereas someone with sciatica will fear chronic troubles. Placebos affect patients and subjects differently, depending upon these and other factors. The circumstances in which pain is evoked or relieved are as important as the kinds of people who have it.

Acute and Chronic Pain

Generally, it seems to me, the pain of chronic disease has been studied more than the pain of acute disease, but pain specialists might not agree. In patients with acute localized muscle spasm, injections of saline into the painful area gave slightly better relief than a local anesthetic, which made the investigators wonder whether they were really performing acupuncture. Many more studies are being carried out thanks to the stimulus of the new Office of Alternative Medicine at the National Institutes of Health.

Within what time limits can we accept any improvement as the result of a placebo? A blood sugar level that falls an hour later seems a plausible effect, far more than levels that return to normal over six months. What to deem a placebo response has bothered investigators since William James. Placebos usually work quickly, whereas organic disease has a slower response to therapy, making it difficult to separate natural history from any long-term benefit of a placebo or a complementary medical practice.

Studies of pain usually record an effect in minutes to hours. If endorphins play a role in pain relief, there may be a quick response and a slow response. We may not be talking about the same thing when we refer to all such responses as the result of a placebo. The clinician usually wants relief that is long-term—days or weeks rather than hours —but we must distinguish short-term from long-term effects if we are to wrest some sense from the placebo response.

Improving Illness, Not Disease

My review of placebo research has convinced me that complaints are helped by placebos, but I find little evidence for objective improvement of diseases. George Bernard Shaw is said to have exclaimed at seeing the pile of crutches and eye glasses at the healing shrine of Lourdes, "But where are the wooden legs and glass eyes?"

Three Kinds of Disease

Diseases fall into three categories: (1) the innocent, which come and go quickly and for which any intervention will appear helpful; (2) the stubborn, which persist for some time and for which intervention may help; and (3) the intractable, which defy medical care yet need treatment most of all. Observers of a treatment trial program should demand proof that a disease that has been cured was in fact present, regardless of how it was helped, especially if claims are made for the success of unusual approaches.

Symptoms are helped in most trials. By their very definition, symptoms must be subjective rather than objective, as with migraine, seasickness, rheumatism, dysmenorrhea, postoperative pain, spinal tap headache, sciatica, and the like. Nowhere have I found evidence that objective improvement in an organic disease has occurred in a placebo trial. Diseases may indeed improve with placebos, but the reports are not convincing except regarding problems like peptic ulcer where improvement is the rule in controlled clinical trials. I take such healing to come from the clinical situation and not from the placebos as such, but others disagree. Warts, after all, do go away with all kinds of treatment. It is also claimed that very low fat diets help unclog coronary arteries, but such studies are subject to overinterpretation and observer variation.

Hypertension brings the dilemma of disease and illness to the fore, much the way irritable bowel does. In anyone, blood pressure can rise with excitement, tension, fear, or other strong emotions. For years experts advised that only sustained high blood pressure counted as a disease. Recently, however, it has become clear that so-called white coat hypertension, the temporary spasm of the arteries that comes when a doctor takes the blood pressure of some people, does lead to permanent hypertension. Claims that one or another hypertension therapy works turn on when contraction of blood vessels becomes permanent and whether anatomical abnormalities can be countered or prevented by various measures. When pathophysiological phenomena lead to anatomical change, it is hard to find convincing evidence that they can be reversed by hope or love or placebos. Many trials of patients on the "verge of hypertension" agree in their findings that weight loss and sodium reduction decrease blood pressure, whereas a more recent analysis by David Eisenberg and colleagues found relaxation more effective than no therapy in reducing hypertension, but not much better than a placebo. The Tessmans, Irwin and Jack, who know statistics, in examining some claims supported by citation, found considerable extension from the data about lowering high blood pressure; unsubstantiated generalizations abound. Not all people with high blood pressure have the same kind of hypertension, in any case.

My claim that placebos affect persons and illness, not disease, raises conceptual problems. Placebos could affect people because of changes in neurotransmitters, which then fill receptors to open or close channels, the brain modulating itself in response and in turn influencing disease. Fright can kill, voodoo can lead to sudden death, and malign influences can affect normal persons. People do fight cancer, die of fear, or keep going until after the wedding, until Christmas, or until they give up.

High blood pressure, asthma, and several other clinical problems may be helped by suggestion, by placebo, by the ceremony of the consultation, by the relaxation response, or by many other nonspecific but helpful approaches. Most behavioral strategies have proven slightly better than no therapy at all, but often they are no more effective than what others might call placebo therapy. I put all those complaints in a functional rather than an organic category, confessing my uncertainty.

In trials of drug therapy for heart failure, however, about a quarter to a third of the patients in the control groups showed improved symptoms and "significant decreases in cardiac output and increased pulmonary artery wedge pressure." We may see changes in function, but I cannot find evidence of changes in disease as measured by structure. Many take hopeful refuge in the recognition that disease is multifactorial, that changing a patient's expectations may change that patient's neuro-chemistry. Reducing stress by maneuvering the relaxation response may decrease the amount of catecholamines secreted and so lessen the likelihood of a cardiac arrhythmia. Asthma can be relieved by reassurance. Suggestion and consolation, hope and laughter, may well prove to have benefit for disease. I hope so.[5]

Neurobiology to the Rescue

In commenting on such problems, William James in 1890 concluded "that a certain amount of brain physiology must be presupposed or included in Psychology. . . . Mental states occasion also changes in the calibre of blood vessels, or alteration in the heart beats, or processes more subtle still, in glands and viscera. If these are taken into account, as well as acts which follow at some *remote period* because the mental state was once there, it will be safe to lay down the general *law that no mental modification ever occurs which is not accompanied or followed by a bodily change.*"

Neurobiological explorations make it possible to imagine that if emotions are programs in the brain, their pathways can be influenced by words, by symbols, by placebos. Neurobiology brings consolation to physicians who demand mechanisms. All sensations change brain function: smell, taste, sight, hearing, and touch are linked physiologically. If the emotions are only a complex arrangement of brain functions emerging hard-wired from the brain, words and symbols should have an effect on physiology, or even on disease, simply because humans are constructed to receive them, our receptors awaiting the right stimuli. The reaction to a disease could prove as substantial as the disease itself. For now, however, I continue to draw an arbitrary line between disease and illness, fearing that I show myself a reductionist.

Precisely because placebos help illness more than disease, they are important to doctors' understanding of their role and how they can help their patients and to our concepts of health and disease. And placebos help to explain the relief that comes from complementary approaches.

Relief comes from placebos, but the evidence for placebo benefit for organic structural biomedical disease remains insubstantial. The gratifying advances in the treatment of diseases, organic problems that can be seen, measured, or photographed, have not been accompanied by equal progress in the management of illness, specifically pain and suffering, which represent 80 percent of the problems coming to most primary care practices. It is that 80 percent who are eased by complementary approaches, Christian Science, placebos, and other therapies. They compose a very large group, and the help provided by such alternatives is very important.

This conclusion is supported by studies that look at whether social and psychological factors have influenced survival of patients with many different cancers. In every case, the biology of the tumor overrides the "potential influence of life-style and psychosocial variables once the disease process is established." However much we dream of the contrary, the evidence tells us otherwise.

What Kinds of Patients Respond to Placebos

About one-third of any group will respond to a placebo. In controlled trials much effort is put into eliminating likely placebo responders, for a successful effort brings far more conclusive results than accepting their presence. Later, doctors will give the active agent on trial to some patients, a third of whom might have won relief from a placebo. The argument goes that physicians cannot predict placebo responders and so must treat everyone. A case could be made for trying the cheapest drug or even a placebo or alternative measures first, depending on the urgency of the clinical situation.

One suggestion unlikely to be taken up is treating ulcer patients with an active drug for one week only, checking thereafter to see whether the ulcer heals as fast as if treatment were continued. I liken this approach to sledding on a hill: if you push the sled over the edge, it should go down all the way, at least as long as the snow lasts.

The Search for a Placebo Responder Personality

Placebo responders cannot be classified by personality, by cultural and socioeconomic status, by suggestibility, or by anxiety level; sex, age, and intelligence do not matter. Such people have been characterized by A.K. Shapiro (1971) as "compliant, religious, hypochondriac, anxious, less educated and frequently using cathartics; disturbed and likely to react to drugs with atypical reactions; anxious and depressed; dependent; ideational; neurotic; extroverted; and so on." Free-floating anxiety, along with stress, are the most likely characteristics believed to predict a clinical placebo response.

No one so far has been able to predict who is likely to respond to a placebo in experimental studies. In one study, depressed and anxious psychiatric outpatients were given a green placebo and asked to note their symptoms over the next hour. Control patients were told simply to spend the hour in a quiet room to see how their symptoms might change. Patients without pre-placebo symptoms had nothing to feel better about, so they showed little change. Patients with mild levels of anxiety improved with any stimulus, but patients with higher levels of pre-placebo anxiety felt worse when given nothing and felt better after taking the green placebo. Suggestion and reassurance obviously helped.

Clinicians recognize the anxious person as the prototypical patient who might benefit from a placebo. The more severe a person's pain, the more likely that person is to respond to a placebo; that is true for dental pain, but not always for psychoneurotic somatization. So-called autonomic awareness, now called visceral hypersensitivity, is an ill-defined concept. It means that some people are just more aware than others of what is going on inside their body. It ought to have some bearing on the placebo response but does not.

Acquiescence must be important as well, for college students with anxiety and depression improved on placebos especially if they were anxious to please. The literature on placebo response in psychotherapy is so vast that I have had to conclude that no single personality type is characteristic of the placebo responder. The context in which the pill is given may be the most important factor.

Nonresponders have been characterized by Shapiro as rigid and emotionally controlled; they are "rigid, authoritarian, stereotypic, tend to use the mechanism of denial, and are not psychologically oriented."

Informing the Patient

Not much is known about the effect of a placebo on patients who have been told that they are getting a placebo. Fifteen newly admitted neurotics were told, "Many people with your kind of condition have also been helped by what are sometimes called 'sugar pills,' and we feel that a so-called sugar pill may help you, too. Do you know what a sugar pill is? A sugar pill is a pill with no medicine in it at all. I think this pill will help you as it has helped so many others. Are you willing to try this pill?"

A week later, thirteen of the fourteen patients who took the pills were improved, with a 41 percent decrease in symptoms overall. There are problems in generalizing from this study of neurotic patients, however. They had already undergone a one-hour interview, which presumably brought its own benefits, and there was no control trial for either drug or interview. The authors were not sure whether the placebo treatment was a form of psychotherapy or whether the benefits came from the patients' faith in the therapist. This important study suggests that placebos can work even when patients are told the truth about what they are receiving, which is how I began this book.

Common sense might tell us that persons with a dependent personality, with faith in others and particularly in physicians, are more likely to be relieved by placebos than someone more withdrawn and skeptical. Or that acquiescent people, anxious to please, will be convinced that they have less pain in a way that might not happen if they were sitting at home taking pills all alone. The placebo response may be inconsistent in any one person: a woman may respond with relief after delivery but not on another occasion.

The placebo responder personality has not been well defined as yet.

Not everyone responds to placebos, but why is hard to explain, especially if the mechanisms are in place in our neuroendocrine analgesic systems. What is there about some people that makes them good placebo responders?

Some years ago medical students were given placebos described to them as either stimulants or sedatives; they were not told which. They were then given pink or blue capsules. Thirty percent of them noted drug-induced changes; sedation occurred six times more frequently than stimulation. Blue capsules were more likely to produce sedative effects than pink ones, and the more capsules a student took, the more pronounced the effect. This suggestibility of sophisticated, if anxious, medical students reminds us of how careful we must be about placebo responses. Circumstances will vary, and the reversion to an infantile state when people get sick surely must enhance the likelihood of a placebo response. The placebo response is greatest when anxiety is great and when pain is severe.

Most of us will be helped by a placebo at some time or other, a testimony to our common humanity, to most people's need for community and friends in time of troubles. Most men and women are not lone wolves.

Pain is paramount among the complaints relieved by a placebo, and relief of pain and suffering is a common reason for patients to seek out doctors. For the clinician, pain needs a sharper definition than the simple one of "I am in pain."

What Is Pain?

Pain was defined in 1979 by an official body dedicated to its study, the International Association for the Study of Pain, as "an unpleasant sensory and emotional experience associated with actual or potential tissue damage or described in terms of such damage." Most mainstream doctors think of pain as rattling along the neural fibers like a train from New Haven to Grand Central Station; if we can derail or sidetrack the engine, the patient will suffer no more. Doctors are troubled by patients with chronic pain, whether in back or belly or head, and have come to recognize how well antidepressants relieve such pain. Even as we accept the mantra that such agents put the serotonin back in the neural cleft—which is a scientific description of why pain goes away—specialists search for the site of pain in whatever bodily orifice or organ they know the best.[1]

Acute Versus Chronic Pain

The same word, pain, is used for acute pain as for chronic pain, but the two are quite different. The line between them is set by experts at six months; acute pain usually involves tissue damage, whereas chronic pain—pain that lasts longer than six months— often lacks that objective evidence.

Acute pains follow well-tracked neural connec-

chapter seven

Patients

and Pain

tions, some of which go upward to the brain to bring the pain into consciousness and some of which trail downward from the brain to inhibit pain at its source. Chronic pain is more enigmatic; its origin is often elusive. I think of acute pain as having modulators, whereas chronic pain has no modulators, only translators of the sorrow that has no vent in tears. To modern science and technology chronic pain offers a stern reproach. Theologians find meaning in pain, and martyrs bathe in it, but doctors—gastroenterologists, anyway—are versed more in scatology than in eschatology. Unfortunately, chronic pain is something doctors often think people should be able to snap themselves out of. In *The Body in Pain*, Elaine Scarry wrote, "To have pain is to be certain; to hear about pain is to be in doubt." That message should be on the wall opposite every doctor's desk, where he or she can see it every day.

Pain as Punishment, Pain as Sorrow

An old practitioner advised us medical students to ask patients with chronic pain, "What have you done that you should be punished in this way?" and suggested putting a hand on the patient's knee to lessen any harsh inference. Joking he may have been, but his meaning was clear: all of us, doctors and patients alike, sometimes cast blame for what has happened, assuming that under the cover of pain are hidden shame and guilt.

"Punishment" is the first definition of *pain* in the *Oxford English Dictionary*. *Pain* often seems to be a word that patients use to gain their doctor's attention when they really mean another kind of suffering, what some call existential pain, with no obvious locus. C. S. Lewis, the famed British theologian, got it right: "Pain has two senses . . . A) A particular kind of sensation, probably conveyed by specialised nerve fibers . . . [and] B) Any experience, whether physical or mental, which the patient dislikes." Pain in the latter sense, he adds, is synonymous with "suffering, anguish, tribulation, adversity, or trouble"—a definition the doctors ignore.

Doctors argue about whether pain originates in the periphery—that is, in the arm or leg or wherever it is felt—or whether it skips the spinal cord and is interpreted in the head, matters discussed later in this chapter. The benefit that comes from antidepressants, those serotonin re-uptake inhibitors, supports the notion that pain is perceived at the center, that is, in the brain. Mind-brain and spirit are as important in how we bear pain as the body, for mind and spirit join suffering to chronic pain.

The opposite of pain is not pleasure, for as someone suggested, pleasure is satisfied just to be. Delighted with the sensation, no one looks for its cause. In contrast, someone suffering from pain looks to stop it or at least to relieve it. The opposite of pain is numbness, not pleasure.

Pain has only four letters, but it discovers saints as well as sadists. In a wonderful meditation on pain, Culture of Pain, David Morris brings us Saint Sebastian, eyes fixed tranquilly on Heaven although his body is pierced by arrows; he should be writhing in pain, but his serenity emphasizes the dilemma of where pain is perceived, in the central brain or in the peripheral nerves. Hoping for eternal bliss, the saint suggests how pain can be modulated and interrupted. The psychoanalyst Carl Jung knew that: he advised physicians to reframe the problems of their patients to help them find a meaning in suffering, even if that meaning lay in the cross they had to bear.

Doctors often discover a relationship between martyrs and patients with functional disease. Functional complaints have been more common among women than men; that may come from circumscription of women's lives that until very recently left them with no outlets beyond motherhood and the home. When I was writing this chapter, a young businesswoman came to me complaining of dyspepsia and bloating that had begun on Mother's Day several years before. It turned out that she had been moving up the executive ladder of a local firm, but shortly before the pain came upon her, she had decided that her place was at home with her two children. That may have been coincidence, but I doubt it, just as I doubt that it would have been helpful to eradicate any baleful H. pylori bacteria from her stomach.

Morris tells of another young woman with the chronic pain of a mangled leg. "With a cane and a heavy metal brace . . . stiffly, awkwardly" she walked to the pain clinic. Doctors suspected that the source of her pain lay deep "within the flesh, beneath thick layers of scar tissue," leaving the reader to wonder whether she had been a dancer or a beautiful woman regretting her lack of wholeness. Her lingering pain—translated bitterness?—surely came from more than just the C-fibers in her leg.

Sex has connections with pain, as both the Marquis de Sade, who gave us sadism, and Leopold Sacher-Masoch, who provided its willing victims, knew. To understand that, one has only to scan advertisements in local throwaway newspapers that glorify pain and sexual arousal. Others look for the origin of pain, and many other human troubles, in repeated abuse in childhood, but do not always ask whether the abuse was real or imagined.

As Ivan Illich, a well-known social commentator, pointed out, the trouble with treating pain is that the whole problem of pain has been taken over by physicians and medicalized "as a systemic reaction that can be verified, measured and regulated. Only pain perceived in this objectivized form constitutes a diagnosis that calls for a specific treatment." The pain that doctors act upon is different from the grief, guilt, sin, anguish, fear, hunger, impairment, or discomfort that may be translated into pain.

Many commentators suggest that chronic pain is wordless, but I take it to be not so much wordless as a cry in a foreign language. A pain is a sign, a computer icon opening a file full of sorrow. Pain does not always run along those C-fibers. To treat chronic pain with anodynes is to mistake its translation.

The Pain Patient

The patient with chronic pain, known in medical jargon as the pain patient, casts the problems of pain into sharp relief. Practitioners know implicitly how important the patient is in determining the response to any disease or injury and how much a seemingly minor problem will disable some people. One person will keep working with a bad cold that would put another to bed for a week. Hypochondriacs are well known to laypeople and physicians alike; such perpetual invalids were known to the Greeks. In The Republic, Plato speaks of Herodicus, a physician who "by a combination of training and doctoring found out a way of torturing first and chiefly himself, and secondly the rest of the world . . . by the invention of lingering death; for he had a mortal disease which he perpetually tended, and as recovery was out of the question, he passed his entire life as a valetudinarian; he could do nothing but attend upon himself, and he was in constant torment whenever he departed in anything from his usual regimen, and so dying hard, by the help of science he struggled on to old age."

The apparently healthy patient wrapped up in pain that defies explanation is surely different from the patient with pain from pancreatic cancer, as severe as any pain can be, who persists in work and in life, as the late Cardinal Bernardin of Chicago showed so bravely. People perceive and interpret pain in different ways, not all susceptible to a simple neurological interpretation even when one cause is cancer. The physician may detect and evaluate disease objectively, but patients know their pain even if they cannot always interpret it.

Acute pain is not all bad, for it calls attention to something that demands treatment. In contrast, F. D. Hart calls attention to the "little martyrs." "The patient with a chronic pain that cannot be shaken off has to learn to live with it and to evolve spiritual complexities to make it tolerable. . . . Relatively few patients with chronic pains ask their physician for death and deliverance, and very few commit suicide." For them, "Pain is spelt with a capital letter and is truly an old friend. . . . This is not a medical or psychiatric problem, but a social one that concerns the personality. Here the Pain is not just an old friend but an essential part of the sufferer's existence: it is not so much a part of, as a partner in, the sufferer's life." Chronic pain becomes a companion, like another person. There is, of course, a high prevalence of depression in patients with chronic pain, with the usual arguments about the chicken and the egg.[2]

Most physicians recognize how different can be the responses to pain. In *The Puzzle of Pain*, Ronald Melzack commented: "Pain, we now believe, refers to a category of complex experiences, not to a specific sensation that varies only along a single intensity dimension. The word 'pain,' in this formulation, is a linguistic label that categorizes an endless variety of qualities" (Melzack 1973). Pain is not a single experience that can be specified in terms of a defined stimulus. Pain, like sight and hearing, is a complex perceptual experience influenced by the unique history of the patient, by the meaning he or she finds in the pain, and by state of mind. He goes on, "In this way pain becomes a function of the whole individual, including present thoughts and fears as well as hopes for the future." Many new aspects of the physiology of pain perception provide further evidence that the placebo response lies mainly in the brain.

Melzack, who with Patrick Wall fathered the "gate" concept that I will shortly discuss, has now expanded his conception of pain. He proposes that in the brain there is a *neuromatrix*, genetically endowed but shaped by continuing sensations from the periphery. The neuromatrix provides a sense of the body-self and is responsible for the interpretation of nervous impulses as pain: "Warmth and cold are not simply 'out there.' Only temperature changes are. The quality of warmth is a function of the brain, not of the degrees Celsius." We might wonder whether Melzack's concept of the neuromatrix parallels the mind or represents the site of spirit.

Doctors uncomfortable with pain as more than sensation coming from those nerves labeled C-fibers must learn the difference between pain as sensation and pain as perception. Writers have known that for a long time: "This new pain of yours, for example, what word suits it best? Throbbing? Beating? Lashing? Burning? . . . It's not one word. Pain has to be a little story. It has rules. A little story that starts with 'like . . . the leather knife of a shoemaker. . . . A mirror shattered into a thousand pieces in your body, like the ice that will form. . . . Like the sharp little stones that pierced your body when you were a child' " (Shalev).

Visceral hyperalgesia, or "altered sensory perception of visceral sensations," is the fancy biomedical term for why some people are more sensitive to their internal workings than others. Many learned reports try to explain "regional manifestations of increased excitability of spinal neurons"—what common sense would take as responses to fear or anxiety. In the end, such researchers may find mechanisms, but not causes. The poets know better.

Pain and Culture

Thanks to medical anthropologists, doctors have come to learn that people from different traditions deal with their pains and aches in dramatically different ways. Couvade offers a dramatic example: in some societies the husband of a pregnant woman climbs into bed to groan with pain while the woman, quite calmly, bears their child. From time to time, a man will tell me of his nausea when his wife was pregnant; I usually take this to be a clue to the psychic origin of his dyspepsia.

Cultural backgrounds have well-known influences on pain perception: first-generation immigrants of Mediterranean origin reported pain at levels of radiant heat that northern Europeans described only as warm. Fifty years ago, descendants of the English pioneers proved more stoic in reaction to pain than newer arrivals. Jews wanted to know what caused the pain, whereas Italians were satisfied with its relief. Their grandchildren, however, suffer headaches, bellyaches, and backaches in the same way as the descendants of the Pilgrims, which tells us how important culture is to the sensation of pain.

In addition to past experience of pain and cultural factors, the meaning of the situation and how much attention is paid to it—which involve anxiety and suggestion—are important in determining how much pain one feels as well as the responses to the pain.

David Morris summarizes the biocultural perspective on pain: (1) pain is more than a medical issue, far more than nerves and neurotransmitters; (2) pain has historical, psychological, and cultural dimensions; and (3) the meaning that the patient brings is fundamental to the experience of chronic pain. In focusing on the social and cultural more than on the unconscious and psychiatric aspects of pain, Morris ignores some unconscious determinants, but he calls attention to how conflict, stress, and emotional trauma transform what might be only a local injury in one person into apparently endless torment.

Pain Relief Systems

Two distinct but interwoven systems relieve pain: (1) a *neurological* network, highly organized and complex; and (2) a *hormonal* supply of endogenous opiates that permeate the body. As more is learned, the unified nature of neural and hormonal systems should become apparent, but for now it is convenient to think of them as separate but equal.[3]

The Neurological Network

Small nerve fibers, the famed C-fibers, carry pain impulses, but their perception can be inhibited by larger nerve fibers that run alongside the small nerves to the spinal cord. The small nerve fibers that account for pain perception can be activated by many stimuli, from heat to the chemical mediators of inflammation; the more frequent the stimuli, the more readily pain is felt.

The sympathetic nervous system also has a role in pain perception, but the exact mechanism by which its injury leads to the unpleasant sensations called causalgia will not concern us. Secretion of catecholamines, especially serotonin, is important and underlines the explanation of why antidepressants are such effective pain relievers.

A mechanism in the dorsal horns of the spinal cord acts as a gate, increasing or decreasing the flow of impulses from peripheral C-fibers to the central nervous system. The large fibers act at the spinal cord to close the gate to inhibit the perception of pain. Stimulation of these fibers may explain the effectiveness of massage or acupuncture or even counterirritants. Whether the major contributions are nervous or hormonal, or—more likely—mixed, they provide one plausible mechanism by which placebos might influence pain perception.

Running from the large fibers that inhibit pain by closing or lowering the gate, other pathways lead to a central control area in the upper brain. That in turn influences, through descending fibers, the modulating properties of the spinal gating mechanism. This central control trigger may open or close the gate, raising or lowering the threshold for pain. The important point is that the gate is raised or lowered "in terms of prior experience" *before* the system responsible for pain perception and response is activated. "The gate control theory also suggests that psychological processes such as past experience, attention, and emotion may influence pain perception and response by acting on the spinal gating mechanism. Some of these psychological activities may open the gate while others may close it" (Melzack 1973).

The central nervous network of the brain monitors, perceives, and changes the perception of pain. Feeling pain is more than a stimulus-response reaction of the outmoded specificity theory, which held that a specific pain receptor in the skin responds to a painful stimulus with a one-to-one relation between the receptor, the size of the nerve, and the nature of the painful stimulus. Yet when patients complain of pain in the arm or belly, or elsewhere, too many physicians still look for a single point source that will yield to a single therapeutic intervention regardless of what they know about the gate theory, about endorphins, and even about the paramount influence of higher brain centers on the perception of pain. Recent evidence suggests that tissue injury evokes long-term changes in the brain that contribute to the sensations of pain and that set up a memory of pain that can be activated by otherwise inconsequential stimuli. The amino acid glutamate plays an important role in all this.

Pain is more than just the sensation felt. How one feels *about* the pain is as important as how one feels the pain or its intensity. Painful stimuli simultaneously influence both sensory processes and emotional processes, presumably by midbrain circuitry, which is so crucial to how pain is felt.

Stimulation of discrete sites in the brain also raises the threshold at which pain is felt. The degree of pain depends on the intensity of the stimulus, but the processing of pain and its interpretation is vitally dependent on psychological processes. These affect the *pain threshold*, which is the intensity of the noxious stimulus necessary for a person to perceive pain, as well as *pain tolerance*, which is how long it takes for someone to recognize a stimulus as pain. Beecher summarized the pertinence of the placebo in this regard. "The great power of the placebo provides one of the strongest supports for the view that drugs that are capable of altering subjective responses and symptoms do so to an important degree through their effect on the reaction component of suffering."

Hormones

The healthy body tries to maintain a constant state: blood sugar and mineral levels are kept within a very narrow range. When they are altered, compensating mechanisms come into play. When the serum sodium level falls, for example, the healthy kidney stops excreting sodium until the normal level is restored. Fever helps stop infections; even so, bodily reactions try to bring the body temperature back to normal.

It comes as no surprise that pain also triggers a system for its own relief. Severe pain stimulates endogenous analgesic systems but then neutralizes them once they are activated. The reader can think of morphine as relieving pain, and of pain as counteracting the effects of too much morphine; that must be why people who have taken an overdose of a sedative are kept awake and walked around. Wakefulness may provide the physiological antidote to sedation, just as pain gives the physiological antidote to analgesia, and numbness is the metaphorical response to pain.

Inflammation carries its own surcease. Opioid peptides are generated by immune cells in the nerves of inflamed tissues to make up an endogenous pain-relieving system that blocks pain from the periphery. Morphine injected into the knee joint in amounts so small as to have no general systemic effect relieves postoperative knee pain quite effectively. Generally, pain can be relieved by smaller amounts of opioids when they are used to prevent pain rather than to abolish it, and the same holds true in the periphery: blocking pain locally before it worsens gives more relief.

Many old-fashioned remedies, such as mustard plasters and turpentine, and even rubefacients, such as Vicks VapoRub, must have brought much of their benefit by stimulating such local peripheral opioid receptors, just like touching or massage.

Opiate refers specifically to any product of the opium poppy. The effects of most such naturally occurring products are counteracted by naloxone, a remarkably helpful antidote to narcotic overdosage. Opioid is the term for any compound, natural or synthetic, whose effect in the body is counteracted by naloxone.

Naturally occurring opiates relieve pain by inhibiting its neurotransmission; presumably membrane channels of cells are opened or closed. Fortunately, such knowledge is not essential to understanding possible placebo mechanisms. Opiods and opiates, generated endogenously or given by mouth or injection, fit into natural opioid receptors in the brain, gut, and elsewhere to bring pain relief. A certain intensity of pain stimulates the waiting endogneous opiate systems: mild pain is less effective in revving up the system than more intense pain. This makes sense because pain is a warning system; one that let us ignore a hot stove, for example, would be more harmful than helpful.

Endorphins are normally occurring opiates found throughout the body. Some direct measurements of endorphins in cerebrospinal fluid are pertinent. In one study, patients with chronic pain had endorphin levels half as great as pain-free control subjects, but when pain was relieved by a placebo, endorphin levels in the spinal fluid doubled. Those who got no relief from a placebo showed no change in the levels of endorphins. Placebo responders may have had lowered endorphin levels in spinal fluid to begin with, but more study is needed.

As it happens, such studies should not be taken too seriously, for there are no really accurate techniques for measuring the opioid analgesic systems. Observers take the worsening of pain by naloxone to imply endorphin relief of pain, but some studies suggest that placebos stimulate endorphins, and others that they do not, because they rely upon such indirect assessments. Observers studying dental pain have found that patients who respond to a placebo have more pain if they are given naloxone to inhibit endorphin activity. In contrast, naloxone had no such effect in patients whose pain did not respond to a placebo.[4]

Even if we could measure opioids accurately, we might still fail to understand their release. A blue pill might stimulate a higher level of endorphins than a red one, a pill in the hospital might produce higher levels than one from a drugstore, and so forth. Still, we can already examine the mystery of why one person can help another by prescribing such pills, although we may not be able to explain how. Gottfried Leibniz suggested long ago that if we could stroll through a very large brain, looking at all its circuits, we would still not understand where love or hope or faith reside. The reductionist would counter that on such a stroll we would at least see the circuits blinking.

Mechanisms of Pain Relief

In summary, there are at least three mechanisms for endogenous pain relief, two neurological and one hormonal, all working in concert: (1) areas in the brain inhibit pain perception through descending pathways that control information reaching the brain; (2) neural circuits in the spinal column inhibit pain transmission upward by a local gate that must be partly responsible for relief by acupuncture or counterirritants; (3) finally, opioid circuits, nonopioid pain-relieving systems related to the sympathetic nervous system, and hormones like catecholamines and cholecystokinin play a very large role in reducing pain.

Drugs relieve pain in different ways. They (1) block the transmission; (2) stimulate suppressive pain mechanisms; or (3) work centrally to make patients indifferent to pain. Agents like aspirin, acetaminophen, and the nonsteroidal anti-inflammatory agents block transmission from the periphery. In contrast, opiates like morphine and codeine act centrally on the brain to activate pain-suppression mechanisms.

Placebo Analgesia

It seems highly likely that attention and perception are where placebos work. Endorphins may not provide the sole mechanisms, however, for endorphin stimulation should provide global generalized pain relief, and this is not the case. That is, placebo-engendered analgesia should reduce sensation in areas not under study; if it did, pain lessened by a placebo in one hand should also reduce sensation in the other hand, but that does not happen. Endorphin release is probably an effect of placebos, but how they work is still hidden from us. Such observations make it likely that placebos help pain not by local or even general mechanisms but by directing attention away from the stimulus.

Doubtless, several different mechanisms will be found responsible. Analgesia is a very complicated matter: stress makes some people feel pain more readily, whereas it makes others ignore it.

Someday it may be possible to characterize the healing personality, but knowing that one healer stimulates endorphins better than another may not explain that one physician is more effective than another. One patient may generate more endorphins than another, but such measurements will do no more than help us glimpse the mechanism. We already know the remarkable feature of pain relief—the triumph of the placebo—that one person can help another simply by trying.

Expectancy seems to be where placebo relief lies. Humans differ from animals in looking to the future: the expectancy of clinical improvement leads to improvement. This is particularly true with functional problems, like high blood pressure. It may well be that patients should be taught to utilize expectancy. Hope, after all, helps.[5]

Maintaining illusions may provide a key to mental health, a consideration pertinent to the placebo response. Illusions have been divided into three categories: (1) self-enhancement, which means looking back on one's experiences and attributes as positive; (2) an exaggerated sense of personal control; and (3) unrealistic optimism about the future. Taken together, these resemble what experienced psychiatrists have suggested are the clinical benefits of a good prognosis for the individual patient, one that predicts a good result and recovery. The expectations of teachers predict how their students will do: a student whose teacher thinks he or she is stupid will do less well than another whose teacher has very high expectations. All of us have known joyful people whose only memories of their past are happy ones; they do not recall the unhappy events that all must face. Many of these people, my father included, lived on into serene old age. Optimistic expectations may help people live longer and happier lives. That is something that everyone concerned with placebos must keep in mind.

chapter eight

Autonomy

and

Respon-

sibility

Three

Patients

The accounts of Norman Cousins, editor and writer, and Franz Ingelfinger, editor and physician, lie at opposite ends of a spectrum. Cousins celebrated the power of people to heal themselves, an acquiescent doctor in the background, whereas Ingelfinger related the peace that came from letting someone else take care of him, even though he knew more than most about the disease that was to kill him. Editor of the *New England Journal of Medicine*, Ingelfinger opened its pages for Cousins's first account; Ingelfinger's own story was published after his death in the same journal. Although these writers are linked in that way, their lessons are different—as is that of a third patient, whom I shall introduce at the end.

Norman Cousins: A Writer-Patient

In 1976 Norman Cousins gained wide notice with a story of his illness that might have seemed as unfathomable to physicians as the casting-out of devils had it not been published in the august *New England Journal of Medicine*. Cousins's account was widely accepted by people anxious for a clue to self-help and by physicians feeling guilty about their new technological emphasis and prowess.

The Complaint

Ten years or so before, Cousins had developed general achiness and gradually stiffening neck, arms, hands, fingers, and legs. During a very trying hospital admission, he wrote, there was "no agreement on a precise diagnosis," even if there was a "general consensus" that he had "a serious collagen illness." One expert gave him only "one chance in 500" of full recovery. Because I have not read the evidence on which these diagnoses were based, they seem as conjectural as those of a witch doctor. With so lugubrious a prospect, Cousins convinced his physician to give him intravenous vitamin C in extremely large doses.

The rest of the story became a medical classic. To encourage his will to live and the "full exercise of the affirmative emotions," Cousins moved from the hospital into a hotel, where he arranged for old comedies and videotapes to be shown to him. Belly laughter brought him salutary relief, or so Cousins and his physician were convinced. At the end of several weeks of ascorbic acid and laughter, a remission was his reward.

Rational and Irrational Medicine

Cousins's report confirms the difference between rational medicine and the irrational medicine that so dismays physicians thinking about placebos and alternative approaches. Cousins improved, to be sure, but there is little evidence of a cause-and-effect relation between therapy and cure. The reasons that Cousins brought for his therapy are the partial explanations seized upon by popular nutritionists and faddish therapists, a celebration of a possible effect abstracted from a general view. We can always find a reason to do something.

Sidney Kahn puts it well:

> From a profusion of guesses, influences, suppositions, hypotheses, possibilities, speculations, Cousins, by idiosyncratic alignment and juxtaposition, has chosen allergy, adrenal exhaustion, red blood cell clumping, placebo effect, endorphins, Vitamin C, cell oxidation, unknown biochemical effects of the pituitary stimulated by mental processes, etc., to erect a structure that is only one of the several score he could have created just as easily and with equal validity from the same building blocks. . . . We enter the realm of scientism, the use of scientific terminology and date for unscientific purposes, the artificial and arbitrary linear linkage of scientific material to support unjustified conclusions.

Professional Responsibility

Although twentieth-century charlatans also plunder science to supply a rationale for their treatments, it would be hard for a licensed physician to justify such measures without more precise marshaling of evidence. My wife can suggest as large a dose of vitamin C to her friends as she gives me, but as a professional, I have to weigh my advice to others. Cousins's physician allowed his prominent friend to decide upon such therapy, but if Cousins had worked out a rationale for cutting off a finger to cure his malady, I hope his physician would have disagreed.

Psychiatrists tell of a patient fearful of impregnation by the Holy Spirit who lost her delusions when her uterus was removed. Presumably, Cousins's physician decided that intravenous vitamin C was harmless and that it could not worsen an outlook already grim. The outcome was happy, but we do not know whether the remission represented placebo effect, natural history, or a psychopharmacological benefit that demands further study.

Physicians have questioned whether Cousins had any serious chronic disease or whether his illness was a self-limited one that would have disappeared on its own. They have no way of knowing, for no objective account has been published, as far as I know. I wrote to Mr. Cousins asking for some objective data from his physician. He graciously sent me an inscribed copy of the book that grew from his article, but I did not find any relevant data there. I wrote to his physician, but my letter was returned. I have to conclude that the most famous case of self-help in the 1970s remains an account by a patient whose beliefs have had an enormous influence on opinion simply because of his prominence. I interpret his report as an example of a man escaping the frustrations of his physicians and allowing the natural course of events to unfold unimpeded by more diagnostic maneuvers and drugs with their myriad effects—and side effects.

As Florence Ruderman put it, "And this may, very often, be the value of the 'placebo': it frees the patient from other standard or experimental drugs, which may overwhelm the body's defenses, or create diseases of their own—whose harmful effects may be greater than their benefits."

Cousins was lucky to leave the hospital.

Helpful Emotions

Like most other physicians, I conclude that Cousins got better on his own. The movies beguiled him while time passed, but laughter alone did not cure him. Cousins has raised important questions, even if we disagree with his premises. Most physicians probably believe, as Cousins himself recognized, that he was the beneficiary of a "mammoth venture in self-administered placebos." Yet Cousins asked a very important question: "Is it possible that love, hope, faith, laughter, confidence, and the will to live have therapeutic value?" In *The Healing Heart* he suggests, properly, that "laughter was just a metaphor for the entire range of the positive emotions." Later he had second thoughts, which need emphasis: "I never regarded the positive emotions, however, as a substitute for scientific treatment. I saw them as providing an auspicious environment for medical care."

Neal Miller echoed him: "To what extent do laughter, beauty, love, affection, success, or even being able to express anger counteract the effects of stressors, and to what extent do they have an independent positive effect on health?" Very little scientific work has focused on mechanisms that operate in pleasant circumstances rather than in unpleasant ones, almost as if investigators have the idea that the normal human condition is pleasant, and stress is abnormal. What about the chemistry of confidence?

Cousins was characteristically in control of his disease and his therapy at every point: "One of the most tragic effects of major illness is the sense—the realistic sense—of loss of control over one's life, and over one's environment. . . . The seriously ill patient is deliberately rendered helpless, denied control over anything that has to do with his illness or his care." A friend, Priscilla Norton, points out that one paradox in Cousins's account comes in his own singular lack of humor. She wonders whether all those belly laughs brought some balance into a life otherwise serious.

The scientific approach would test the hypotheses clinically by controlled trials and objectively by physiological observations in a behavioral laboratory. An irrational, if empirical, approach would set up clinics and beam the Comedy Channel to hospitals. Unfortunately, there have been serious discussions of the therapeutic benefit of comedy but no rational study. Comedy is amusing and doubtless does not harm unless some broken ribs hurt from laughing. I love the old comedians for the fun they bring, not for their healing powers. Health networks modeled on Cousins's account might alternate nutritionists and faith healers with comedians and physicians, all pitching their own therapeutic programs specializing in the Marx brothers, the Three Stooges, or their modern heirs. (Not Woody Allen, I think. His doubts might make some sick people worse.)

It is useless to meditate too long on Cousins's case; the report is little different from reports of recovery from curses, voodoo, and other magic. We know too little about the original disease. I doubt that the *New England Journal of Medicine* would have published a report of a similar outcome written by a patient less celebrated or by a physician with as little data. Physicians owe each other precise descriptions of such events and all the data.

Patient Autonomy

Cousins's account of his alternative approach raises questions about professional responsibility and the limits of patient autonomy—how much the patient should decide. The widespread view that the primary aim of medicine is to restore personal autonomy means returning patients to where they were before they got sick. Anything more, a whole repair job, so to speak, would put the physician in even more parentalistic a relationship than ever. I may want my physician to repair my coronary arteries or my back, but I might cherish my neuroses. Ivan Illich has reemphasized how much medical practice and physicians have medicalized society.[1] Patients with pneumonia or an ulcer simply and sensibly want to get well. I have never heard a patient ask me or any other physician to restore his or her autonomy. Offered the choice between psychotherapy and steroids for ulcerative colitis, most patients usually opt—as they should—for medicine and leave their autonomy to fend for itself. Physicians and patients work out such matters as they establish a relationship.

Patient autonomy must be weighed against physician responsibility. Too hard and fast a rule of patient autonomy overrides the professional responsibility of physicians. Call it parentalism if you will, but the physician is an expert, licensed by the state to apply special knowledge. It would be a lamentable abdication of responsibility if physicians did not recognize that they usually know more about the disease than their patients. Although physicians have been trying to make patients equal partners in decisions about the patient's health, the equality so much talked about really does not exist in many physician-patient encounters, and it is foolish to pretend that it does—or that it should. A patient is a sick person, often upset and worried, and to that extent the patient is not the person he or she was before getting sick. In working to restore health, the physician cannot always act as if patients are always prudent and equal decision-makers, particularly during an acute illness. The patient needs help, and even during a chronic illness, inequality may exist. Lawrence Henderson put it well: "A patient sitting in your office, facing you, is rarely in a favorable state of mind to appreciate the precise significance of a logical statement. . . . The patient is moved by fears and by many other sentiments, and these, together with the reason, are being modified by the doctor's words and phrases, by his manner and expression." Emotion does not diminish the importance of the patient's story, nor the necessity for the doctor to try to understand what the patient wants, but it highlights the need for medical knowledge and the value of a professional.

One may well ask why physicians should control placebos. It might be possible for patients to give themselves placebos out of conviction, as Cousins did. Before they go to a physician, most people have tried home remedies, most of which are at least partly placebic. Once the physician is consulted, however, professional responsibility will play a deciding role. Alternative-medicine practitioners try to bridge the gap.

Franz Ingelfinger: A Physician-Patient

Franz Ingelfinger, an expert in diseases of the esophagus, ironically enough developed cancer of that organ, so it was natural for all his doctors to assume that he knew more than they about what to do. Later, the question arose whether Ingelfinger should be given radiation or chemotherapy. Because of his knowledge and because he was editor of the premier general medical journal, his doctors asked him what he wanted them to do, and in addition many medical friends sent much contradictory advice. "As a result," said Ingelfinger,

> not only I but my wife, my son and daughter-in-law (both doctors), and other family members became increasingly confused and emotionally distraught. Finally, when the pangs of indecision had become nearly intolerable, one wise physician friend said, "What you need is a doctor." He was telling me to forget the information I already had and the information I was receiving from many quarters, and to seek instead a person who would dominate, who would tell me what to do, and who would in a paternalistic manner assume responsibility for my care. When that excellent advice was followed, my family and I sensed immediate and immense relief.

Ingelfinger—scientist, editor, and physician—had to turn decisions over to others who would be loyal to his best interests, however those might be defined. Ingelfinger was articulate and, to the end, able to express what he wanted. In his own medical world he was far more powerful than Cousins, and the doctors taking care of him had good reason to understand what he wanted and to fear that their reputations might depend on how well he fared. That is not always the case, and in the name of autonomy obscure people may suffer because they are less able to say what they want or because their physicians are less willing to listen.

A Laborer-Patient

Well-intentioned equality can lead to bad results if physicians do not sometimes affirm their own superior knowledge, as in the following anecdote.

In praise of physician-patient equality, a well-known ethicist told how, when young, he let an old man die rather than force him to submit to diagnostic procedures that he did not want. The patient was a sixty-six-year-old man, previously healthy, who had pneumonia, confirmed by chest X-ray. When he did not quickly improve on antibiotics, more laboratory studies suggested that a cancer might be complicating the problem. The patient angrily refused further unpleasant diagnostic procedures despite "prolonged pressure" and then began refusing even routine tests. A psychiatrist concluded that he was not mentally incompetent and that he understood the severity of his illness, but that he was making a rational choice in refusing the test.

Considerable disagreement ensued among his physicians. It was clear that "if he survived this crisis he would be able to return to a normal life and would not be an invalid or require chronic supportive care." Convinced that the patient was making a conscious rational decision to refuse a particular kind of treatment, his doctors let him die. His case was presented as a model for patient autonomy: "The intellectual and emotional strength necessary to resist the powers of the medical system to persuade and force him to accept what they wanted to offer must have been enormous. He died a dignified death. . . . I am sadly moved that he had to expend his last measures of intellectual and physical energy in ongoing debate with his physicians" (Siegler).

A physician more sure of his or her professional responsibility might have concluded that a sixty-six-year-old man with pneumonia who had not responded to treatment, with trouble breathing for almost a week, was not in any state to make a rational decision if only because he might not have been getting enough oxygen to his brain through his stricken lungs. He had been well three days before coming to the hospital, with no chronic disease.

Age played a role in the doctor's considerations: "I would have demanded a more perfect 'mental status examination' and would have scrupulously checked a younger patient for evidence of a 'toxic delirium' or an acute depression. . . . I might have acted differently with a younger patient." The medical discussions, with their air of catharsis, leave me unable to recognize the arguments as valid. The attending doctor said, "I readily admit that my clinical judgement that the disease was rapidly progressive and almost certainly fatal further influenced me." Here, the principle of complete autonomy for a competent adult overrode better clinical judgment.

A more appropriate course might have been to have done the necessary procedures—to have treated the patient and faced a lawsuit with equanimity. To the outside observer, it seems that the man was afraid of pain, and instead of negotiating with the patient about his fears and concerns, the stance of patient-physician equality allowed what might have been a curable disorder to lead to death. It is unlikely that a court or jury would conclude that a man restored to health had a valid claim for damages. Autonomy and considerations of equality should have played a much smaller role than they did. Aged seventy-four as I write this, I know that the now older physician has reevaluated the role of age in his decision-making, and his confession has taught us all.[2]

Equality for the patient is balanced by the physician's professional integrity. Authority has to stand for something. A Catholic physician will not be asked to carry out an abortion, and patient equality meets its limit in what the physician as person and as professional can accept as reasonable.

Moreover, patients are not and cannot always be equal partners. Their interest in getting well is far greater than the doctor's interest in promoting their health. The old adage has it that the doctor who treats himself has a fool for a patient and a fool for a physician. If that is true, as we doctors all profess, patients are less likely to make adequate choices unless guided by a physician. Ingelfinger and Cousins portray different sides of this problem. We should continue to tell such stories and to ponder them.[3]

Beneficence to the Rescue

The pendulum is swinging. To balance the shortcomings of the patient-autonomy ideal and the medical parentalistic habit, David Thomasma emphasizes the importance of beneficence, acting for the benefit of another and responding to a plea for help. He also takes into account the values of the physician who must make choices in the care of the patient. In a sense, by avoiding the imposition of values or decisions made in the best interests of the patient without the patient's participation, both physician and patient respect their own values. Thomasma reawakened the notion of the importance of moral character in educating physicians. I believe that physicians must be more than passive guides: they have the expertise and training to help the patient choose the best way, as the patient sees it.

Objections to placebos come on largely ethical grounds. Most ethicists flatly disapprove of placebos, whereas physicians are a little more likely to approve of their selective use to benefit patients. Ethicist refers to someone, usually a philosopher, who thinks about what is right and what is wrong, or at least what is better or worse. The term parallels *physicist* and is intended to convey the same relation to ethics that the scientist has to physics. In medical practice *ethicist* now means one of those people who evaluate how doctors act with patients but who themselves rarely take care of patients.[1]

Truth-Telling and Lying

Most ethical objections to placebos come on the basis of truth-telling, for thirty years a recurrent theme in biomedical ethics, especially in considering the dying patient dominated by the parentalistic physician who withholds facts to control the situation. The sharp light cast by the question "Should dying patients be told the truth?" bleaches out the chiaroscuro of the placebo picture. Curiously, I have not seen many objections from ethicists to some outrageous claims of alternative practitioners.

The Dying Patient

For a long time well-meaning physicians shielded their patients from the depression that they were sure would follow news of impending death. Leo Davidoff, a noted neurosurgeon, was typical.

> If the patient has a very malignant tumor, I tell the relatives that a tumor was found and

removed. . . . Whether the patient is told or not will then depend on what he wants to know. The questions and answers may be something like this:

Patient: "Well, Doctor, how did it go?"

Doctor: "Fine, fine, everything went very well."

Patient: "Was everything removed that doesn't belong there?"

Doctor: "Yes, it's all out."

Over the years since the 1950s most physicians have come to agree that dying patients or any patients with a potentially fatal illness should always be told the truth. A vast literature has grown up around this tenet, and Richard Cabot of Massachusetts General Hospital, Boston, has been enshrined as its American apostle.

A formidable clinician and teacher, Richard Cabot was careful to emphasize that a true or false impression can be conveyed without words.

Now, I was brought up, as I suppose every physician is, to use what are called placebos, that is bread pills, subcutaneous injections of a few drops of water (supposed by the patient to be morphine), and other devices for acting upon a patient's symptoms through his mind. . . . It never occurred to me until I had given a great many "placebos" that, if they are to be really effective, they must deceive the patient. . . . Suppose we said to him: "I give you this pill for its mental effect. It has no action on the stomach"; would he be likely to get benefit from it? No, it is only when through the placebo one deceives the patient that any effect is produced. It is only when we act like quacks that our placebos work. (Cabot 1978)

Cabot argued, like many others, that patients who get pills for one complaint will expect pills for other complaints. He told the following story. "This poor woman complained that she had a lizard in her stomach, that she felt his movements distinctly, and that they rendered her life unbearable. Doctor after doctor had assured her that the thing was impossible, that no such animal could subsist inside a human being, that the trouble was wholly a fanciful one, and that she must do her best to think of it no more. But all such explanations and reassurances were of no avail." Then a physician told her that he could give her a chemical that would dissolve the lizard, which would then be excreted by the kidney. That physician gave the woman methylene blue dye, which gives a deep blue color to the urine: "The woman took the medicine and perceived to her amazement and delight that a blue color was imparted to her urine, recognized that the lizard must have been dissolved, and was at once free from all her symptoms."

Cabot went on to tell how the symptoms recurred, "another lizard grew," and the patient "turned up at still another Out-Patient clinic under the charge of a very honest physician, to whom she told her story. . . . He found that she had an excess of gastric juice in her stomach, the irritation of which gave the gnawing and scratching feeling which she attributed to the presence of a lizard. Having discovered this fact he proceeded to treat her for this trouble, which he succeeded in curing, and after that time the lizard never grew again."

Cabot must have been the very honest physician of his tale, but we do not know how long his follow-up lasted. Measurements of gastric acid have proven of so little diagnostic value that modern clinicians long ago gave up measuring it. Cabot substituted faith in measurement for fear of a lizard.

I imagine that the woman's cure was short-lived, but the confrontation between her beliefs, probably of European peasant origin, and those of the high-minded Boston physician is wonderful to contemplate. To relieve his patient, Cabot imposed his own system of beliefs with his therapy. In Chapter 10, I discuss the role of lizards in folk medicine to suggest that Cabot's patient was not as bizarre as modern physicians might think.

Cabot comes down against placebos and for telling the truth in all circumstances. Indeed, he was the founder of the CPCs, educational exercises in which a doctor discusses what he or she thinks might have been wrong with a patient, and afterward, the pathologist gives the "correct" answer found during the operation or in the autopsy. His book *The Art of Ministering to the Sick*, written with Russell Dicks, then chaplain at Massachusetts General Hospital, has been a guide to me for fifty years, one which I reread from time to time and which I have recommended over and over again to medical students. Cabot's strictures on lying, however, seem self-righteous, even sanctimonious.

Some years ago, I read an account of Richard Cabot and Hugh, his brother, both graduates of Harvard College and its medical school. A skeptical professor of surgery at the University of Michigan, Hugh is quoted as saying, "There are fools, damn fools, and then there is my brother Richard." Richard's positive nature and absolute certainty made him an ideal teacher. He must have had a lot of common sense, for about high blood pressure he wrote elsewhere in 1947, "Those who are subject to unavoidable financial or domestic worries and those who have to earn their living by muscular work usually succumb within a year or two."

Richard was not always as right as his subsequent canonization might suggest. He endorsed a program of laxatives and cathartics for the treatment of drug addiction, a program characterized by others as "diarrhea, delirium, and damnation." He believed in celibacy, and his marriage was proudly celibate.

More important for his insistence on always telling the truth is the story of another brother, Ted, who, in the days before insulin, was slowly and painfully dying of diabetes. "Ted, his parents, and Richard agreed that Richard should act to end his suffering. Several days before the appointed time, Ted said a goodbye to his mother which she described as 'enough to live on and live by for the rest of her life.' He struck a note in this farewell, she said, 'that brings all life and death itself into perfect harmony and to be with him is to be with God' " (Ward).

Ted was thirty-two, Richard only twenty-five, when they made the awesome decision that Ted should die on November 10, 1893. We can only wonder how much Richard Cabot's later insistence on absolute frankness came from the need to justify that decision to kill his brother. We can only conjecture that his insistence on telling the truth to the dying represented a lifelong attempt to turn his act into a model for others.

Hans Zinsser, his contemporary, wrote that "a well-known American physician who was at the same time—to my mind—a canting moralist held on occasion that absolute, uncompromising truthfulness is the only justifiable position, however cruel." He added: "The truth can be exaggerated when the doctor talks to a hopeless patient. . . . One must pick one's situations and one's cases, and adjust the truth to the judgement of wise kindness." I do not want to diminish the message by attacking Cabot, for many of us justify our acts and lives by offering rules that accord with what we prefer. Yet Cabot's story is perplexing.

Truth Versus Reassurance

Telling the truth to every patient has become a greater virtue than mercy. Only a few physicians still weigh the feather of beneficence against this weightier virtue. Dietrich Bonhoeffer warned that " 'telling the truth' means something different according to the particular situation in which one stands. Account must be taken of one's relationship at each particular time . . . in each case the truth which this speech conveys is also different." Sissela Bok gave a different guide: "Whether you are lying or not is not settled by establishing the truth or falsity of what you say. In order to *settle* this question, we must know whether you *intend your statement to mislead*." Marilyn Smith countered that since one's intentions are strictly private, the person lied to will never know your intent. "If I force you to answer whether you are intending to mislead or not, what is to prevent you from further intending to deceive, that is, from lying?"

Keeping the diagnosis from a dying patient is not quite the same as giving someone a placebo. The proverbial prudent man would choose to know that he is dying in order to make final plans; the dying patient is usually harmed by not knowing the approach of death, whatever the emotional cost.

Placebos fall in the category of white lies—common, trivial, not meant to injure, with little moral import. Critics argue mainly against what they lead to: dependence on pills and drugs and loss of confidence in both physicians and bona fide medicines if their recipients find out. But what if they feel better? Others worry that placebos may encourage other deceptions in medicine for benevolent reasons. Arguing against the consequences for others does not imply that placebos are harmful for the patients who get them.

Until recently, physicians were not asked to make utilitarian decisions about social harm outweighing individual benefit. Recently, however, they have been forced into the position of a double agent in the cause of reducing medical care costs by forgoing tests or referrals to subspecialists and so saving money.

Complimenting someone on a tie or a dress or a lecture keeps the social machinery oiled. Common sense should also help separate the trivial from the important. Reassuring a patient who must undergo an emergency operation that everything will be all right is not the same as telling a father of six with gastric cancer that he has only a little ulcer.

"You are a doctor in the emergency suite. A young man has come in with a liver ruptured from an automobile accident, and as he is being wheeled to the operating room, he asks, 'Doc, will I make it?' What would you say?" That is a story I tell medical students, college students, and physicians. I have come to expect that college students, like first-year medical students, will choose strong reassurance, but that fourth-year students and physicians will be more mealymouthed, offering something like "I hope so" or "We'll do our best." Even a recent ethical column criticized my strong plea for doctors to give reassurance.

In a famous contract law case, *Hawkins v. McGee*, read by all law students in the United States, where it is known irreverently as the "hairy hand" case, Dr. McGee tried to repair Hawkins's scarred right hand with a skin graft. After a long and troublesome postoperative course, Hawkins claimed that surgeon McGee had guaranteed a very short recovery: "Three or four days, not over four; then the boy can go home and it will be just a few days when he will go back to work with a good hand."

Since then, law students have wrangled over whether McGee had made a promise or just offered good-hearted reassurance; the uncertainties of medical practice make it impossible for a physician to give the warranty of a commercial contract. Most seem to agree that physicians should not be held liable for simple human reassurance. The rare times when the courts have upheld a suit for a contract to cure have involved egregious and self-seeking claims by physicians about what they can do for their patients.

Truth-Telling and Autonomy

Patient autonomy, with its origins in the civil rights movement of the 1960s, carries over into the medical relationship adversarial preconceptions that physicians are trying to put something over on patients. That is no model for physicians or patients. The truth can be couched in hopeful terms. Denial brings comfort, and not everyone can handle unvarnished truth. Cousins asks, "Is it possible to communicate negative information in such a way that it is received by the patient as a challenge rather than as a death sentence?"

Liberty may have its limits, and the current valuation that puts autonomy ahead of health may not last forever. Patients in chronic pain are rarely the same people they were: someone with cancer, kept alive by tubes in vein and gullet, dependent on others to turn from side to side, confused by a long hospital stay, is not the same person as when in good health, and is unlikely to make the same decisions that might have been made before.

Doctors have to respect even the helpless patient's decisions, asking permission, talking over what to do and what not. But it is impossible for physicians to assess the decisions of patients when all they can do is nod or grimace. That is why living wills and the durable power of attorney have gained popularity: to ensure that someone we trust to be loyal to our best interests, to the choices that we have made when we are in our full power, will make decisions about us when we are unconscious or deranged.

Nor is the patient in pain the same as he or she was without pain. Enhancing autonomy requires relieving pain and only then talking of long-term goals. Over and over again physicians hear, "You are the doctor. You decide." They take that acquiescence to be the universal condition of the sick, not the claimed autonomy they read about. It makes them agree on professional beneficence.

For physicians, telling the truth may mean telling the truth to themselves, that a patient is dying and that they should not prolong the dying. The matter grows poignant in the young patients with AIDS, particularly those abandoned by friends and family or those for whom, in just the opposite way, the family wants everything done. A resident in medicine, Eric Krakauer, has described the staff's reaction to turning off the breathing apparatus for one young man whose family had agreed to let him die, and had left while the patient was gasping for breath. "Nurse N sat down at the bedside, took Mr. K's hand, stroked it gently, and spoke soothingly to him. Tears ran down her face. I stood behind her with my hand on her shoulder, fighting back my own tears. Mr. K's gasps became less frequent and violent. After 30 or 40 minutes, they ceased altogether." The young physician recognized only too late that the patient had not received adequate doses of morphine to prevent slow suffocation.

Illness or disease weakens control over the body, and it has been likened to increased gravity. As Lisa Newton puts it, "The body, usually transparent, suddenly becomes opaque. It takes on weight; where before the arm was weightless, reaching for the book it now is heavy."[2] Physicians try to restore control over the body to their patients; not until after that do they worry about more abstract notions.

Strong and Weak Parentalism

Arguments against placebos often bring up paternalism, now better called parentalism. Physicians used to feel proud about taking charge, but now they are usually attacked for it. Parentalism is defined as an action taken by one person in the "best interest" of another without the explicit consent of the person to be benefited. Strong parentalism is an action taken against the expressed wishes of a patient, to save life. A classic case tells of a young athlete, burned beyond hope of ever playing again, who kept saying that he wanted to die but whose life was saved against his will. He is now a lawyer battling for patient autonomy. Weak parentalism, more common, is an action taken by a physician in the best interest of a comatose patient on the presumption that a physician knows best what a comatose patient would decide.

Not telling a patient how placebos might work seems different from strong parentalism. There are good arguments for telling the truth.[3] Physicians usually don't know enough about the patient to predict that telling the truth will result in depression, which not even a personal psychiatrist can always foretell. Withholding the dire prospects from the parents of a defective newborn to spare them the misery or guilt of making a decision once was quite common, but physicians have no duty to minimize harm to the family, only to their patient. Nor do they have a right to make decisions about someone else's moral or spiritual life under the guise of what is feasible.

Physicians need not always know; indeed, it is sometimes in a patient's interest not to try to find out what is going on beyond the assessment that nothing serious is wrong. Warning against outright lies does not put placebos in the same category as deceiving patients about a serious illness or about their outlook.

Philosophers' Conclusions

Even though Plato permitted lies to the sick and dying, Bok seems reluctant to leave room for placebos as altruistic deception: "1) Placebo should be used only after a careful diagnosis; 2) no active placebo should be used, merely inert ones; 3) no outright lie should be told and questions should be answered honestly; 4) placebo should never be given to patients who have asked not to receive them; 5) placebo should never be used when treatment is clearly called for or all possible alternatives have not been weighed."

My friend Howard Brody compares a physician using placebos with a magician fooling an audience. I disagree, because the physician hopes to relieve pain or suffering, whereas the magician deceives for pleasure. The audience pays, knowing that "it's all smoke and mirrors," whereas patients come for relief. He is right, however, that "healing comes not from the lie itself, but rather from the relationship between healer and patient, and the latter's own capacity for self-healing via symbolic and psychological approaches as via biological intervention."

Others disapprove of placebos for legal and ethical reasons, pointing out that they deceive patients and give them false beliefs; some leave room for placebos in more trivial circumstances. Vitamin C is possibly good for a common cold, and they excuse prescribing it on the grounds that it is without obvious harm.

Physicians' Conclusions

Most physicians of an earlier time, because of their clinical experience, had no problem with the benevolent deception of the placebo. Henderson, a Harvard Medical School scientist, speaks for them:

> A patient sitting in your office, facing you, is rarely in a favorable state of mind to appreciate the precise significance of a logical statement. . . . The patient is moved by fears and by many other sentiments, and these, together with reason, are being modified by the doctor's words and phrases, by his manner and expression. . . . Above all, remember that it is meaningless to speak of telling the truth, the whole truth, nothing but the truth to a patient. . . . If you recognize the duty of telling the truth to the patient, you range yourself outside the class of biologist, with lawyers and philosophers. The idea that the truth, the whole truth, and nothing but the truth can be conveyed to the patient is an example of false abstraction, of that fallacy called by Whitehead "the fallacy of misplaced concreteness."

Dealing with real patients, doctors have used placebos for their symbolic value. "Deception is as integral to the placebo as copper is to bronze. Should we not accept the pragmatic view and in good conscience continue the judicious use of the invaluable placebo?"

One physician divided placebos into those that "build-down" and those that "build-up." The first is confrontational—"You have nothing wrong with you if a placebo helps you"—whereas the second is a gift that "says something that words cannot say at one particular moment." The second placebo may help to form a group, patient and doctor in alliance, which, after all, is one therapeutic goal. "It is the net effect of the health and hope the physician can offer the patient that justifies the special relationship between the two. Nothing but the truth would prove a miserable medicine. . . . What deception is necessary for the prescription of a placebo cannot be judged right or wrong without a situation assessment of the desired outcomes" (Phillips).

For practicing physicians, the real problem comes, as one has suggested, because "ethicists deal with generalizations about problems and fail to take into account that it is always dangerous to apply a generalization to a particular situation. The moment of truth for the doctor is when face-to-face with a person in trouble. To generalize about individuals and prescribe identically is obvious nonsense."

Physicians must apply different remedies for different persons. Giving placebos, like shading the truth, needs to be considered in relation to individuals. In a long philosophical tradition, ethicists sometimes regard the rider on the bus as very much like themselves, which may not always be true.

Jay Katz, a psychiatrist passionate about truth-telling, asks the question in a more helpful way.

Should placebos be left to faith-healers and should physicians instead swear allegiance to new gods of science? Put another way, should physicians extend their assistance to all "suffering" humanity or only to that group which they can treat with their scientific knowledge? . . .

If placebos have a place in the practice of medicine, the physicians must appreciate more fully that placebos are not innocuous, that they can do much harm; for example, by becoming a means for hurriedly doing something in order to see the next patient, when nothing, except careful explanation, need be provided; by not allowing the healing power of nature to take its course and instead prescribing active "placebos" which can produce iatrogenic ailments that require further treatment; by making persons through placebo treatments dependent on physicians, confirming them in the status of patients when instead their "recovery" could have been accomplished through reliance on the person's own recuperative powers; by blinding physicians to recommend with enthusiasm remedies of no value, and disregarding in the process less detrimental alternatives.

On the other hand, too great a restriction on the use of placebos may interfere with care.

Physicians and ethicists should continue the conversation, even if they never completely agree. The empathic physician who emphasizes individual relationships and knows how much patients vary in their needs will continue to use placebos, however much ethicists censure that approach.

Economic Objections to Placebos

One argument against giving placebos emphasizes the expense of paying for "inactive" drugs. Millions of dollars are spent on inadvertent placebos and placebic medicines, but, as I have emphasized, many procedures for reassurance are also placebos: the results of the procedure will surely prove negative, and when I tell the patient that the test is normal, his or her anxiety will be relieved, and that in turn will lessen the pain.

Indeed, treating many complaints first with active drug or placebo and investigating only those patients who do not improve might reduce the cost of medical care. A major problem might come in deciding how much to charge for a placebo, but against that cost must be put the much larger cost of diagnostic investigation, plus the inconvenience or discomfort of the procedure. The relief that comes to physician and patient alike when pain is assuaged by a simple exchange is easy to reckon.

A stronger argument can be made against the use of impure placebos, drugs effective for one disorder but used for another. Ralph Nader has claimed that more than six hundred available drugs are no more effective than a placebo, and noted that over a billion dollars' worth of prescriptions have been for drugs considered ineffective by the FDA. Such drugs cause side effects, and although they assuage the physician's feelings, they bring more harm than good, as I have already noted.

Diagnostic Objections to Placebos
Masking Disease

Critics worry that placebos will relieve pain of a serious origin, so that a disease which might have been treated goes unrecognized until too late. That gives placebos more credit than they deserve, for there is little convincing evidence that a short diagnostic delay worsens the outcome of most diseases, except in malpractice courts.

I am not sure that earlier detection of disease in a person without symptoms leads to a better outcome.[4] Many people are sure that it does, but medical evidence is not so convincing. Placebos help, but I have found little or no evidence that placebos are powerful enough to delay for very long the manifestations of any disease; if such a delay ever proves very long, the power of placebos will deserve even greater admiration. A delay of a few weeks to await the effect of treatment usually does not injure the patient's prospects for recovery. Physicians may have taught the lessons of early detection too well. Placebos help pain and lessen suffering, but they do little to relieve the serious manifestations of organic disease.

Many symptoms should never be put off with placebos. No competent physician would deal with sudden abdominal pain by other than emergency diagnostic tests and even an operation. But chronic abdominal pain is another matter. Other complaints that require speedy investigation include rectal bleeding, chest pain, or any acute pain, regardless of its site. That is why a physician is needed to decide when placebos may be useful.

Detection Bias

There is ordinarily no sharp line between when a disease begins and when it can be detected. What looks like a life span prolonged after early detection of a problem may be just the result of detecting it at an earlier stage than before.[5] For example, a rare form of liver disease, primary biliary cirrhosis, used to be a disease of middle-aged and elderly women; it ran a short and fatal course because it was not recognized until late. Specific blood tests now allow its detection in young women, years before they develop symptoms. The patients with the disease are no longer old women with jaundice and itching but much younger women with no complaints at all, except that knowing about their disease has made them more attentive to symptoms.

Therapeutic Detours

A strong argument against placebos holds that even if placebos work, they may block the efforts of patients to get at the cause of their problems by seeing a psychiatrist, or at least adjusting to life's problems, and by developing self-help procedures. Psychiatric help may prove so wrenching, expensive, or unpredictably beneficial that, weighed in the balance, trying a placebo in some people may seem easier.

People often deny illness or disease as long as possible. A patient who has finally screwed up the courage to seek a doctor's help and who gets a placebo may not return, telling anxious relatives, "The doctor said I'm OK." This is another risk associated with placebos.

It is true, too, that a pill which brings relief, even if it is a placebo, may accustom the patient to look for a magical potion for every problem. Here, there is no easy answer. Giving placebos could promote drug-taking and dependency, but procuring some prescription or other from the doctor has such a long history that it seems improbable that the tendency or desire can be strengthened any more. The popularity of over-the-counter medicines shows how widespread is faith in pills. Placebos add only the proverbial drop in the bucket.

Placebo as Nocebo

Some argue that placebos can cause real harm, turning into nocebos which harm because of (1) unintended side effects, like those of antibiotics, or (2) conditioned responses from any previous bad experiences. This belief in the dark side of placebos has been used as an argument against fully informed consent, for explicit suggestion of possible adverse effects may lead patients or subjects to look for and find them. "Informed consent may be hazardous to health."

The person who worries too much about the rare complications of a medication may not be in a positive enough frame of mind to mobilize the healing processes of the body. This intuitively sensible suggestion seems plausible.

Malpractice and the Placebo

Patients might react angrily to finding out that they have been given placebos, particularly when they have not been helped. "You mean," the patient might say, "you gave me a sugar pill and charged me for your services? What kind of fool do you take me for?" It is not easy for me to imagine giving a professor of molecular biology at Yale a sugar pill for his or her pain without explaining what I am about. Otherwise, anger, resentment, or hostility might well lead to a lawsuit or at least to a change of physician.

If giving placebos were to become widespread and well known, uncertainty about the medical profession might grow. Even if physicians gave placebos only in a helpful, parentalistic spirit, patients who were not helped might react angrily.

I have used placebos as a symbol of communication, for contact with the patient. In our litigious society, however, the only placebos likely to be tolerated for general use will be the impure ones that take some action that can be credited with treating the ostensible source of trouble. Few physicians now give the sugar pills that the previous generation provided, but they do give antibiotics or vitamins or other injections to reassure patients. More rely on diagnostic tests or operations, knowing that reassurance comes in many forms.

Lawsuits

Curiously enough, there have been few legal rulings on the use of placebos and the risk of a malpractice suit that doctors run by prescribing one. In the past, the placebo aroused little interest among lawyers, probably because most patients never found out about them, so case law based on precedent and judicial decision has not been erected.

So many links now exist in the chain between physician and patient that the placebo transaction is sure to become known and the patient to sue for deception, fraud, or even malpractice unless the physician has been forthright beforehand. As more physicians practice in groups, and team medicine becomes the norm, giving a patient a placebo is unlikely or impossible to be kept secret. Pharmacists are increasingly unlikely to hide what the customer is getting, particularly when a third party, such as a cost-conscious HMO, is paying the bill. Indeed, an important task is to explore the legal position of placebos. Today more than a few doctors are willing to accept placebos or something like them as harmless, but they are afraid that using them may open the door to legal liability.

In Jurcich v. General Motors, a suit about continued back pain, the court ruled that prescribing placebos was a recognized treatment. Apparently a physician said, "No. You never tell anyone if you are going to give them a placebo; then you know it won't work. You are hoping that you will fool him." The court did not believe that taking placebos worsened the plaintiff's pain, nor did the pain come from the defendant's wrongful act in giving him placebos. Nor was there evidence that the patient had suffered a monetary loss as the result of the placebos. The trial court's ruling was upheld in the appellate court.

That was back in 1976. Whether courts would be as understanding today may be wondered. Reasons for suing physicians who prescribe placebos without telling patients have been enumerated by U. B. Kapp; fraud, informed consent, injury, and breach of contract are the chief issues. Let me take them up one by one.[6]

Patients might sue a physician on grounds that they would have gone to another physician if they had known their doctor was prescribing a placebo. They charge fraud, but judges have commented that malpractice would have provided stronger legal grounds, for it is hard to prove damages that can be recompensed by money, as is requisite in a fraud case. No one, so far, seems to have discussed the question of whether giving an impure placebo, one with some pharmacological action, however irrelevant to the complaint, might provide a defense.

Third-party payers, who have to underwrite the cost of placebos that they might judge worthless, could conceivably sue, particularly if the pharmacist charged more than a minimal amount for the drug. In a unique twist, drug users who have been given inactive powders instead of illicit drugs have threatened to sue for fraud.

More likely grounds for suit might be found in the lack of informed consent when a placebo is given without telling the patient. The problem in winning such a suit, however, lies in showing that harm came to the patient taking the placebo.

A successful malpractice suit for injury would be likely only if the patient had suffered a negative placebo reaction, which is unlikely. Still, claiming that the use of placebos delayed more appropriate treatment might lead to a successful suit. Kapp suggests that a liability is created by physicians who give placebos and so discourage patients from seeking more adequate care. The physician who gives a placebo that relieves the patient runs very little risk, but if the prescription does not help, the physician might well be held liable. The physician or institution dispensing placebos as part of a clinical trial is presumably protected by the original informed consent laying out the double-blind nature of the trial. But once the outcome of the control study becomes clear, ethical and legal considerations demand its end even when its continuance would make the statistical basis stronger.

Breach of contract, the implied promise by the physician to be honest, Kapp suggests, provides only a relatively weak basis for a malpractice suit.

Defenses

The first and doubtless the strongest defense against a legal attack for prescribing a placebo lies in the claim that no damage has occurred because no injury followed. Unless the patient can prove an adverse reaction to the placebo or a worsening of the complaint while taking the placebo, damages will be difficult to prove. The courts, however, have occasionally held precisely that opinion.

If other physicians use placebos, there is no negligence involved in prescribing one. Instead, it is accepted practice.

And because placebos alleviate the complaints of many patients, they are permissible under the doctrine of therapeutic privilege. If a physician believes that telling the patient about the placebo prescription would complicate or hinder treatment or upset the patient enough to cause psychological harm, treatment without informed consent has been held permissible, largely in emergencies; once the patient has improved, full disclosure should take place. To avoid a possible suit, the physician should consult with a colleague to secure an independent written agreement, which seems impractical. A friend has asked whether he should call the consultant while the patient is dressing before prescribing a placebo. Of course, just getting that second opinion might itself have placebo effect.

Solutions

A patient may waive rights to all information; such a waiver can be implied by demeanor, facial expression, behavior, and the like. A waiver of information need not be explicit, but this idea probably needs more study and testing in the courts.

A patient can contract with the physician to withhold information: "You are the doctor. Tell me what I need to know. I trust you, and if you don't want to tell me something that you think will hurt me, don't. I am in your hands." That sounds like an explicit rephrasing of the old-fashioned, once implicit physician-patient relationship.

For placebos in controlled clinical trials, we must ask whether a patient who has a stroke while taking a placebo during a trial has the right to sue the doctor, the organization running the trial, or society. If a drug is shown to reduce the risk of a stroke by one-third in a high-risk group, should all the patients who are controls be compensated, or only a third of them, and, if so, which third?

A patient who receives a placebo during a drug trial loses the benefit of an effective currently available drug and may have been thereby injured. Patients whose ulcers bleed because of a placebo might argue that had they known of the potential consequences, they might not have joined the trial. Yet such trials are needed. One solution might be to pay persons who take part in them because they are serving the public good as much or more than their own. Yet the difficulties of deciding upon the amount of compensation seem very great.

Most arguments against placebos from the patient's standpoint involve one or more of the following: (1) self-determination (not being lied to, not being deceived); (2) economics (paying for "useless" drugs); (3) education (being trained to think that doctors are all-powerful and that pills are necessary for every complaint); and (4) diagnostic delay (any pill or placebo may delay the appropriate diagnostic events so that the patient will grow sicker). In the next chapter I examine what kinds of patients with what kinds of problems respond to placebos in a predictable way.

Mainstream medicine has rightly achieved such canonical status that few remember that it once had to compete with a whole covy of alternative approaches. Paul Starr has described how the Flexner Report of 1910 eliminated most other systems of practice and so facilitated the hegemony of scientific medicine.

chapter ten

Alternative

Medicine

More recently, alternative medicine has found a welcome in mainstream medical practice, especially in primary care, although the term *complementary* is more fitting for what should be a tributary to the mainstream. Homeopathy, one form of alternative medical practice, has grown in fashion partly because its practitioners take time to try to understand their patients and, in that way, heighten the anticipation so fruitful in the placebo response.

Alternative practices are nothing new. H. H. Goddard observed in 1899 that ''cures by mind-cure exist, but are in no respect different from those now officially recognized in medicine as cures by suggestion. . . . We have traced the mental element through primitive medicine and folk medicine of today, patent medicine, and witchcraft. We are convinced that it is impossible to account for the existence of these practices, if they did not cure disease, and that if they cure disease, it must have been the mental element that was effective.''

Most of us can be helped by someone else. When we are sick, we may want more help than when we are healthy, and we are likely to be more receptive to consolation. Any therapist or healer who can establish a comforting relationship with a patient by taking the time to listen, regardless of any theory behind what he or she does, will lighten the patient's perceptions of the problem. That relief makes assessing the objective evidence for alternative medical practices difficult.

Definitions

Alternative medicine usually refers to forms of therapy, most of which focus on mind-body relations that do not fit into current mainstream medical practices. Perhaps "focus" is misleading, for that is not always the explicit aim, even if that is what observers credit. Physicians who practice alternative medicine prefer to call it *complementary medicine*, which has a less adversarial tone, but old habits die hard. Alternative medicine means any therapeutic program that defines itself as outside mainstream practice and that aims at relieving symptoms in some unconventional manner. Sometimes alternative therapy is given by laypeople and sometimes by practitioners who are not physicians; more often, it is given by physicians who practice in a sometimes unconventional manner.

Among the alternatives to high-technology drug-based medicine we find hypnosis, acupuncture, homeopathy, herbal medicine, faith healing, and many other approaches, which I will discuss in the next chapter. Witchcraft and voodoo fall into that category; even if used to make a well person sick, they bring echoes of nocebos.

One major distinction between complementary and mainstream medicine lies in the expressed aim of alternative practitioners to treat the whole person rather than just a specific symptom or a disease.

Holistic implies working with the whole person and is still used to describe alternative practices, but the adjective is not as widespread now as a decade ago. The term had its origin in a book, *Holism and Evolution*, written by the South African prime minister and World War II leader Jan Christian Smuts, who derived the word from the Greek *holos*, meaning "whole." His book is said to be an indictment of reductionism.

Alternative practitioners aim at health rather than sickness. Many mainstream practitioners also treat the whole person, but for the most part they focus on disease, a focus sustained by the triumphs of scientific medicine duly celebrated by professional organizations. The increasing use of term *mind-body medicine*, a translation of *psychosomatic*, suggests that orthodoxy may be yielding to forms of complementary care.

Banished so long from the medical lecture, spirituality, too, has now made its return; even dieticians incorporate such references in their nutrition counseling, but so far they have refrained from ascribing sacramental status to their menus.

What is conventional in one culture may be unconventional in another; acupuncture offers a well-known example. Medical practices differ even from one Western country to another.[1] Germany, France, and the United States all have different popular diseases that it is almost unpatriotic not to believe in. What in France goes as a *crise de foie* ("liver crisis"), in Germany often masquerades as cardiac insufficiency or low blood pressure; in the United States dyspepsia and heartburn are popular maladies. One rejoices to learn that "gas" is a common complaint in Arabic countries, with their generous pools of underground oil and natural gas.

Some alternative medical activities may look irrational, but they should be seen as part of the continuing challenge of the romantic to the rational, which brought the Counterenlightenment after the Enlightenment and, in our time, the postmodern after the modern. The postmodern plea for diversity and pluralism has had much to do with the growth of alternative medicine. Many well-informed people with cancer seek out unorthodox practitioners who emphasize nutrition, personal responsibility, and an improved mental attitude and who provide more personal warmth and support than their more technically oriented colleagues.

Health, Wellness, and Healing

Health

Health has been defined rather exuberantly by the World Health Organization as "complete physical, mental, and social well-being and not merely the absence of disease or infirmity." Until we have done away with disease and infirmity, however, doctors might do well to concentrate on their patients' diseases and illnesses.

I avoid the term *health care*. Public health measures are important: clean water, vaccinations, and quitting cigarettes have all reduced the death toll. Whether physicians give health or just try to cure disease by medical care, I am not certain. I prefer to think that health, like grace, comes from the Creator.

Wellness

The emphasis on maintaining health and wellness (the word is often spelled with a capital *W*) has generated a new movement, found now in HMOs and in hospitals to encourage enrollment. That movement aims at what has been called salutogenesis—in contrast to pathogenesis —but runs the risks of solipsism. If people focus their energies solely on what goes on within them and in their immediate space, they are likely to ignore social, economic, and other factors in disease. Disease is far more complicated than even its depiction in the biopsychosocial model. The wellness movement downplays physiology in a psychological reductionism reminiscent of Emile Coué's old mantra "Every day in every way I'm getting better and better." It also runs the risk of blaming the victim for any sickness: it is hard to have cancer, but it is worse to be blamed for it. Moreover, the narcissism engendered leads to health fanaticism.[2] Economic motives, whether the business of supplying foods and medications for wellness acolytes or the motives of HMOs in cutting costs, all play a role in proselytizing for wellness.

As I contemplate the legion of joggers rushing by my porch with pained expressions, I wonder what they are running from and what they are running for. Doctors can teach prudence and good public and personal hygiene; they can even council against destroying health; but despite all the hoopla, doctors really cannot do much, so far, about keeping people healthy. Reassessing lifestyle and priorities may be an important reaction to disease or illness, but physicians for the most part can act only as catalysts.

Such skepticism does not accord with the recommendations of panels of eminent physicians usually blessed by the federal government and now by many HMOs. Yet anyone watching the swings of what is acceptable and admirable must have doubts about the enthusiastically global assumptions of public health experts and holistic leaders alike.

Healing

At a conference in Hawaii several years ago, I listened with awed delight to a man who declared himself a Buddhist-Methodist preacher. As he talked of healing his patients, I marveled that so many of them had ended up in a pine box, until I realized that he was using *heal* in its spiritual sense, rather than a more physical one.

According to the *Oxford English Dictionary*, *heal* means "to make whole or sound in bodily condition; to free from disease or ailment, restore to heath or soundness; to cure (of a disease or wound)." Another, more figurative definition from that same volume is "to restore a person from some evil condition or affection (as sin, grief, disrepair, un-wholesomeness, danger, destruction); to save, purify, cleanse, repair, mend." The differences resemble the important distinctions between the meanings of *pain*. Clearly, proponents mean quite different things when they talk about healing.

Healing is a term often encountered in nonmedical circles, but it is not a word that mainstream physicians very often use. Healing affects illness only. In *The Healer's Art*, Eric Cassell writes: "I used the word 'healer' and suddenly saw that I had no idea what it really meant." He recognizes illness as the reaction to disease, modulated by culture and psyche. Doctors sometimes cure disease, whereas healers help illness. For Cassell, disease can turn adults into helpless, fearful children; but omnipotent, somewhat magical figures can give them confidence to build a bridge from the world of the sick back to the world of health. A confident, charismatic healer returns control to the sick, gives permission, like a parent. "The doctor's sense of omnipotence is an important part of his function as a healer, something he cannot disown. But omnipotence, like all magical gifts, is double-edged and dangerous; it can strengthen as well as harm its possessor and its receiver. The doctor's feeling of omnipotence can foster dependency, making a despot of the doctor and a child of the patient, or it can give the patient courage to learn control and free himself from fear."

In *Persuasion and Healing* Jerome Frank finds healing to encompass "measures which combat anxiety and arouse hope," which strengthen a sense of self-worth. For him, religious healing shows "the profound influence of emotions on health and suggests that anxiety and despair can be lethal, confidence and hope, life-giving." Both these physicians echo the problems that mainstream doctors have in using the term *healing*: healing affects illness only. If psychosomatic medicine is ever reborn as that aspect of medical practice which looks at the whole person, clarifying what is meant by healing will be an essential first step toward its incorporation into mainstream practice.

Healing indicates claims that modern physicians are loath to set for themselves, with implications that physicians seldom wish to avow. For physicians, *cure* is a more comfortable word because it pertains largely to disease. *Healing* brings a connotation of curing from within, as in "the wound heals," a self-healing return to wholeness that means more than physicians think they can claim: "I dress the wound; God heals it."

Healing, broadly defined by its adherents as "making or becoming whole," rests on five points: nature's self-repair, suggestion, the therapeutic personality of the healer, the expectant faith of the patient, and "an interchange of energy" between healer and patient. As R. Sampson puts it, quoting a holistic practitioner, "To the extent the therapist is able to envision and call forth healing and wholeness within his patients, he is manifesting in action those qualities that are within himself." Healing has more to do with spirit than with body.

That people sometimes do not die but keep living until after a holiday or a birthday, as Bernie Siegel rightly points out and as David Philips has demonstrated, may be telling us something about what hope, belief, and the will to live are all about. Siegel tells his patients to make every day count; learning how to live, some would add, is learning how to die. He has very useful things to say about life and living with cancer or other debility, but I wish that there was less emphasis on the anticipation—or is it only hope?—that mood changes might sway the course of a disease like cancer.

Transformation

Healing refers to ways of strengthening inner resources and the inner self so that the quality of life improves, even when the progress of a disease like cancer has not dramatically halted. It helps; otherwise, the group therapies so popular with psychiatrists and now with the managed care industry as well would not flourish. People do teach one another how to cope; prayer may not prolong life, but it brings peace. For many it is like Pascal's wager: it can't do any harm to believe in God, so why not? Prayer brings solace, and meditation has been credited with more than a mainstream doctor can believe, but these practices surely can bring peace of mind.

Michael Lerner, a layman who has given a lot of thought to such matters and who remains rightly skeptical about claims of miracles, describes the essence of healing very well. "Healing . . . starts within your own mind and body. The capacity to heal is what you bring to an encounter with illness. . . . There are psychological factors as well. Do you believe that your inner-healing resources could make a difference? Do you want to fight the battle?"

People use the term *healing* in so many different ways, and agreement is so unlikely, that the word *heal* is best left to nonmedical practitioners, even though physicians have begun to understand the mystical combination of mind and body that it captures. In reviewing the claims for complementary practices, we need to keep these different usages in mind. We ought to be talking about transforming—changing what cannot be cured—instead of healing.

Growth of Alternative Medicine

Where the high Victorians looked with disdain on stories of miraculous cures as coming mainly from isolated and mountain areas, today's middle-class city people, educated and apparently sophisticated, are likely to turn to alternative forms of treatment.

Alternative medicine practitioners are widely sought after in the United States. Several years ago, it was reported by Eisenberg and colleagues that 34 percent of patients had tried at least one alternative medicine approach and that 425 million visits were made to alternative medicine practitioners, at a cost of 13.7 billion dollars, of which more than 10 billion dollars was *not* repaid by insurance companies. Figures in Canada and Europe confirm that acupuncture, homeopathy, herbal medicine, and massage are widely employed. Presumably, when insurance companies are willing to pay for such therapies (and this is now happening on an experimental basis with Dean Ornish's program to help coronary artery disease), we will be able to regard them as proven, at least to hardheaded, bottom-line-minded businesspeople. And, as I have noted, HMO officials have learned that alternative practices are welcomed by their clients. AT&T now offers the option of acupuncture to its employees, as does Kaiser-Permanente. In my own state of Connecticut, some health plans offer a network of alternative care practitioners to their patients—presumably the high utilizers already mentioned—without requiring physician referral. The cost of this benefit, which assures free visits on a deductible basis, adds 2-3 percent to the annual premium.

Now only a leaky, semipermeable membrane separates alternative practices from mainstream orthodoxy. Alternative institutional and group activities and products, such as conventions and publications, are beginning to mimic the mainstream standards. Several journals have appeared, including the *Journal of Alternative and Complementary Medicine* and *Alternative Complementary Therapies*. Even the American Medical Association heralded its Conference on Physicians' Health in 1996 with the headline "Uncertain Times: Preventing Illness, Promoting Wellness," formerly the battle cry of the fringe.

Alternative medicine has shaped mainstream medicine and helped to define it. In the nineteenth century homeopathy forced mainstream physicians to define their own activities; the advances in medical science came in handy as a way to heighten professional status.

Alternative medicine practitioners refer to mainstream medicine as biomedicine because many of those advances were modeled on the treatment of infectious diseases and trauma, leaving chronic conditions less comforted. The indictment is too sweeping. The aims of alternative medicine are congruent with those of mainstream medical practice because, I repeat, so many complaints have their origin in social, emotional, and economic problems. Mainstream physicians, who largely adhere to biomedicine—let me adopt that term for this chapter at least—may yearn for the magic bullet that will provide a cure for each disease, but mainstream doctors are all moving in the same direction, although at different speeds.

Effectiveness of Complementary Practices

In current medical literature, a movement in mainstream practice called pathography, part of the postmodern movement, gives center stage to the patient's account. That movement recognizes no distinctions between illness and disease, a division that has been so helpful here to my understanding of how placebos help people. Many writers, like Oliver Sacks, proudly praise anthropologists who take the patient's account at its own valuation, but mainstream practitioners and teachers must try to maintain the occasionally fuzzy distinctions between illness and disease. In pathography the distinctions are not important, for what is of interest are not facts but feelings. For that reason, alternative practitioners claim that no satisfactory control trial will ever be possible, for no two patients are alike or need the same treatment.

The effectiveness of alternative medicine will be judged by orthodox medical science in its own ways, usually with the evidence of controlled clinical trials. Such trials are far from infallible: results from one year are often toppled by findings from the next, and the ensuing dissension and statistical squabbles can resemble the arguments of medieval theologians. In proposing a more magisterial approach, I once suggested that asking a panel of seasoned clinicians to try to disprove the claims for a new drug might give as much understanding more quickly and cheaply than the standard controlled clinical trials. That suggestion was laughed away as antiscientific; the mainstream medical world will doubtless continue to rely on controlled clinical trials.

The Office of Alternative Medicine (OAM) at the NIH was established a few years ago, in 1991, under congressional pressure, to evaluate alternative treatments and to help integrate those that were effective into mainstream medical practice. The dissension that accompanied its first few years led the original director, Joseph Jacobs, a Yale Medical School graduate and a pediatrician of Mohawk and Cherokee descent (presumably to guarantee a wider viewpoint), to resign after two years. Although since then, Jacobs has been heard to define alternative medicine somewhat breezily as "things not taken seriously by the medical profession," the Office of Alternative Medicine has more diplomatically characterized as an alternative therapy any medical practice or intervention (1) that does not have sufficient documentation in the United States to show that it is safe and effective against specific diseases and conditions; (2) that is not generally taught in medical schools; and (3) that is generally not reimbursable from third-party billing. The OAM offers six major categories: (1) diet/nutrition/lifestyle changes; (2) mind-body control; (3) traditional medicines and ethnomedicines; (4) structural and energetic therapies; (5) pharmacological and biological treatments; (6) bioelectromagnetic applications.

The responsible advisory group has many pressures to resist, from some functionaries of the NIH who view alternative medicine with disdain and from those who want to be sure that funding goes to the proposals they support.

Whether it is necessary or financially feasible for that office to explore every nook and cranny of alternative medicine's attic needs discussion. In 1995 the OAM provided thirty-thousand-dollar grants to evaluate some of the therapies, from nutrition, health education, lifestyle modifications, and biofeedback and relaxation techniques to acupuncture and acupressure, homeopathy, herbal medicine, chiropractice, massage, antioxidant therapy, bioelectromagnetic therapies, and more. More standard research methods are needed to convince mainstream professionals, although many mainstream researchers are surreptitiously taking antioxidants themselves. Critics worry that publicizing grant awards in the news gives alternative medicine an unwarranted probity, a view that the new chief of that office has publicly acknowledged by admitting that serving on official panels can seem to be a seal of credibility.

What Are the Alternatives?

That all therapies, from acupuncture to coffee enemas, are equally helpful is an idea that few mainstream physicians can believe. Touching and massage represent ways for the patient to feel, literally, that somebody cares, and they may represent a form of psychotherapy or just a placebo. The large number of people coming to doctors' offices for whom high- or low-technology medicine has little to offer must account for the great interest in alternative medicine. In Britain more than 80 percent of physicians responding to a questionnaire wanted to explore at least one form of an alternative approach.

The many new immigrants to the United States have brought renewed awareness of cultural issues in medical care. Researchers in cross-cultural medicine explore ethnic concerns and the biases and beliefs of many immigrants, who may not follow medical directions for a whole host of cultural reasons.

Although complementary medical practices have begun to earn the attention of the medical profession instead of its instinctive disavowal, doctors must still look at them as critically and rationally as at the claims for controlled trials of placebos. The popular enthusiasm for the occult now displayed by the frenzy for accounts of angels must be telling physicians to widen their attention and their metaphors of disease.

The alternative health movement has been called a social movement with no coherent program, defining disease and cure any which way and often taking a part for the whole. Massage is good for aches and pains (as we have seen, possibly because it stimulates spinal cord gate mechanisms) and doubtless also overcomes loneliness, but to elevate it to a method of healing may go too far. Looking into the eyes is helpful to practitioner and poet alike, but the claims of iridologists that they discern disease by looking at the iris have no scientific or theoretical basis. Even the Holistic Medical Association has no firm body of knowledge and practice on which its members agree; the association accepts medication and even surgery as therapeutic and does not repudiate conventional medicine, but that is about as far as agreement goes.

By and large, however, alternative practitioners share specific ways of keeping healthy through daily habits, diet, and what used to be called physical culture. Certain philosophical outlooks permeate their practice.

Personal Responsibility

The alternative medicine movement holds patients as responsible for their health as physicians: people are urged to keep fit, to learn to cope with stress, to eat healthy foods and avoid harmful ones, to eliminate pollutants from their environment, and to cultivate spiritual values.

Encouraging self-reliance is a praiseworthy goal. Far too many modern patients have become passive recipients of medical care, vessels waiting to be filled, usually with drugs. They are often better off being active participants in their own return to health. I have told more than a few patients, "The doctors don't seem to be doing much for you. Why don't you try to do something more on your own?" Sometimes I warn patients who have been vainly looking for some explanation of an ache or pain not to complain too much to their doctors lest more tests be done and something found and cut out that could have stayed in place indefinitely. But I do not know if anyone takes that advice.

Distrust

A sustained distrust of orthodox medical practices and technology pervades the alternative medicine movement. Qualms about physicians and their instruments accompany a general skepticism about professionals; enthusiasts question traditional medical practices from a strong adversarial standpoint. The People's Medical Society, for example, has asked physicians to sign a pledge that almost takes for granted that they are not to be trusted.

Folk Remedies

The alternative medicine movement may take on a antiquarian air when it returns to folk remedies. Folk remedies are not necessarily ineffective—to wit, the growing popularity of garlic for so many human ills, from cholesterol levels on. Chinese remedies have custom to support them, but physicians are learning that more than a few contain unknown active ingredients, which come to doctors' attention when they cause liver damage, or worse. When alternative medications prove helpful, mainstream physicians are likely to consider their benefits purely as a placebo response.

Peppermint offers another hardy example. Mints have been considered a digestive aid for years: peppermints are still sometimes served at the end of a meal, and tincture of pepperment used to be given to relieve gas. Studies have shown that peppermint relaxes the lower esophageal sphincter, and in Britain it has been revived as an agent to relieve the unpleasant symptoms of irritable bowel or spastic colon. Old ways are not necessarily bad ways.

Alternative practitioners understand that not all symptoms have an organic basis and that many complaints arise from emotional, cultural, economic, and spiritual foundations. In that, they are wiser than many of their mainstream peers.

The Green Movement

Vegetables and the environment both play a role in alternative medicine, whose adherents share a concern about the environment. Instead of seeing it as a place of comfort and refuge, they can see it as a potentially dangerous source of disease; the vectors can be air or water or electric wires. Fears of the by-products of modern technology are the origin of the "sick building" syndrome and others like it.

Tenets and Attitudes

In summary, the good complementary practitioner sees the patient as a whole person; views illness and disease as a message about bad habits and opportunity to change them; recognizes the very old idea that physicians can help patients by interacting with them; and believes that patients get better faster when they work with physicians to take care of themselves than when they simply do what they are told to do. James Gordon, now professor of psychiatry and a family medicine physician at Georgetown University School of Medicine, in emphasizing how many patients feel their doctors do not listen to them enough, draws on seven tenets for doctors to consider as they treat each patient —a checklist of sorts: (1) psychological issues; (2) relaxation therapy; (3) self-awareness (by this he means that doctors should be more aware of their own biases toward diseases or patients and of the stresses in their own life); (4) nutrition; (5) physical exercise (here he includes tai chi chuan and yoga); (6) group therapy for patients with chronic disease; and (7) alternative medical practices.

Those tenets are what this book is all about, but I take issue with some prevalent attitudes. Physicians can try to teach patients how to remain healthy, but doing so may remain beyond their abilities. Smoking cigarettes has proven deadly to many, like being too fat or drinking too much alcohol or not getting enough exercise. Yet many of us envy those people who eat, drink, and even smoke too much at the funerals of their more abstemious friends. Their genes have something to do with their good fortune, and their good luck reminds us that although we may be able to keep from harming ourselves, remaining healthy is beyond our current accomplishments. Doctors, like the British royal family, do not live longer than other people, even though they are remembered in peoples' prayers.

The former head of the Office of Alternative Medicine, Joseph Jacobs, has summarized the main attractions of unproven cancer treatments. They are considered nontoxic and natural, and they are directed toward stimulating the patient's immune system, not toward eradicating specific disease. Because they are purportedly tailored to individual patients, the patients feel that they are participating in their own care. Many alternative substances are derived from Native American herbal remedies, but other programs include mind-body medicine, the Simonton Method, the method of Bernie Siegel (about which he offers the wry pronouncement that a study "reported no enhancement of breast cancer survival as a result of participation in this program"), and the Commonweal Cancer Help Program. Jacobs is skeptical about the value of unconventional treatments even in enhancing the quality of life, although this claim is usually made. Nevertheless, in suggesting a helpful collaboration between patient and physician, he remarks wisely, "Patients trust physicians with their bodies and also want to trust physicians with their beliefs."

How Placebos Might Work

I discuss the mechanisms by which placebos might work elsewhere (Chapter 13), but a few comments are appropriate here.

Psychoneuroimmunology is immensely popular in academic medical circles these days, as we will see in other chapters. Here William James's comments on mind-cure are still pertinent: "To the importance of mind-cure the medical and clerical professions in the United States are beginning, though with much recalcitrancy and protesting, to open their eyes. . . . The important point is that so large a number should exist who *can* be so influenced [by the mind-cure movement]." Of the mind-cure movement of the late nineteenth century, he remarked that its literature was "so moon-struck with optimism and so vaguely expressed that an academically trained intellect finds it almost impossible to read it at all." Everything goes: what feels good must be good for you, a criterion that permits an uncritical acceptance of almost any approach.

Examining placebos and their effect brings the question into the open, forcing the recognition that it is *not* the ritual nor the pill that has power, but the patient and practitioner who put time and energy into healing. Inert and inactive, the placebo has no power; the miracle comes in one person helping another. The patient does the work while the doctor or the placebo takes the credit.

At a meeting of the Psychoneuroimmunology Research Society a few years ago a measure of disagreement surfaced. Some participants reported immunological responses to emotional states; others studied functional immune measures with arcane numbers. Curiously, at the same time, a news item garnered from doubtless the same meeting described how people suffering from chronic pain found substantial relief from implants of cow cells. Placebo effects were mentioned but not explored.

Doctors and patients have wondered whether HIV and AIDS bear any relation to depression, under the presumption that the mind modulates immune function. So far, findings are much as for other diseases: prolonged depression comes as patients grow sicker, and there is no clear relation between the effect of depression and the rate at which immunologically active cells decline. To date, depression does not directly account for any significant laboratory findings. Most people want to believe in self-help, so this continues to be a fruitful area for research disbursements.

Experiences can be described in many different terms and in many different ways. Alcoholism has variously been defined as a sin, a crime, and a genetically determined disease. Henry James writes that adventures happen to those who can describe them, and that is just as true of illness or disease. Where physicians will point to the genetic abnormalities or anatomic particularities of cancer, their patients will talk about disability, pain, or distress. Some may even describe a tumor as "the best thing that ever happened to me," once they have transformed their troubles into lessons for themselves and others. Whereas physicians turn to molecular biological descriptions, anthropologists and sociologists prefer culturally specific explanations, which offer lessons in how to understand patients and their troubles. One does not always have to bow to a genetic predisposition: thought precedes will, and will can control action.

Sympathetic physicians can help patients with cancer simply by being there to listen to, or just note, the anguish that the patient may or may not express. Whether that sharing specifically influences tumor biology remains unproven: we do not know that emotional factors can cause or prevent cancer, nor that they can affect recurrence. We do know that doctors can improve the quality of life for cancer patients by paying attention to mind and spirit.

Whether placebos or complementary remedies have the power to change the course of organic disease is open to much question. Dean

Ornish points to the lowering of high blood pressure and the shrinking of fatty deposits in the coronary artery as examples of mind over matter, but blood pressure is notoriously variable and sometimes overtreated. His observations on cholesterol deposits have yet to be confirmed, although his methods are now being paid for by insurance companies. Just as it is hard to separate conventional therapy from placebos, or mind from body, so it is equally difficult to separate the perception of disease, which is illness, from disease itself. Where does a headache go when it is relieved?

I may seem to regard alternative medicine much the way I do a placebo. Indeed, any discussion of alternative medicine in a book dedicated to placebos carries its own message. The equation is not one of disdain. Placebos of all sorts bring relief to many people; likewise, the mechanisms by which complementary medicine practitioners help their patients probably have little to do with the specific approach. Alternative practitioners have much to teach mainstream doctors about the time devoted to patients and the discussion of their general circumstances, about the enlistment of the patient as an active participant in his or her care and more. But the claims made for the cure of organic diseases deserve skeptical scrutiny.

The faith of the person caught up in any health movement must help, in the same way that placebos help. Groups strengthen the healing mode. Assuming personal responsibility is good. There is no need for an adversary relationship between alternative and mainstream medical practitioners.

Claims of Alternative Medicine

If alternative approaches are marketed to patients or consumers, it is the responsibility of the FDA and the Office of Alternative Medicine to assure that they are effective as well as safe. As is so often the case, people argue over what is meant by *effective* and whether it refers to complaints or diseases.

A major problem lies in the claims that alternative medicine makes without routine records of observations. A charlatan pretends to possess secrets in the healing arts, whereas scientists develop hypotheses to explain observed phenomena and then plan experiments to test their hypotheses. The charlatan neither tests experience nor changes hypotheses, and that is where, I fear, some alternative practitioners may also go astray. Few discriminate between disease and illness, as I keep repeating. The triumphs of treating illness presumably are the triumphs of changed perception and attention; complementary techniques may be innocent placebo techniques that depend on faith and suggestion. Practitioners who claim that this or that specific method cures cancer, for example, must prove that cancer was present beforehand and that it has disappeared after therapy—biopsy would establish the fact. Predictability is the key.

Another question is whether any form of alternative medicine has some special insights that would not be possessed by any prudent physician or whether its current allure comes from its novelty in a scientific age. In a rational medical-payment scheme that de-centered the technological aspects of medical practice, physicians would be paid as much (or more) for time spent with the patient as for things done to the patient. That is the contribution of complementary medicine—benefit to the illness, not to the disease.

In this regard, two observations are pertinent. As is so often the case, what William James says about these matters is still applicable: "The obvious outcome of our total experience is that the world can be handled according to many systems of ideas, and is so handled by different men. . . . Science gives to all of us telegraphy, electric lighting, and diagnosis, and succeeds in preventing and curing a certain amount of disease. Religion in the shape of mind-cure gives to some of us serenity, moral poise, and happiness, and prevents certain forms of disease as well as science does, or even better in a certain class of persons."

David Owen, a physician and quondam British politician, suggests that alternative medicine could help strike a better balance in medical care: "It is the reassertion of the traditional medical values where a sensitivity to the individuality of the person is a precious part of the practice of the healing profession. The practice of medicine involves the whole person."

Whether holistic approaches, acupuncture, and psychotherapy achieve their ends by the specific techniques credited or because of the time spent with patients remains uncertain. What is done by the therapist to stimulate healing may vary with the patient and with the patient's experiences. Almost 60 percent of people felt much better after attending an alternative medical clinic for such nonspecific complaints as back or abdominal pain, feeling run-down, and headaches that had not been relieved by conventional practitioners. That finding must be telling us that conventional medicine does not adjust or fine-tune its approaches to different people with different complaints. The buffet of approaches that alternative medicine offers gives the patients with specific problems and idiosyncratic experiences tighter control over their own treatment and a wider selection of treatments.

Ironically, the claims of alternative medicine are best attested to by William James himself. William Osler, professor of medicine at Oxford, was James's friend and physician, but when James was sick in 1910, he went off to an unknown physician in Paris, whom he characterized as a quack. He did not ask Osler's advice, just told him he was going. "My anginoid pain has increased during the past year, tho' nitroglycerin stops it like magic. I go to Paris to consult one Dr. Montier, whose high frequency currents have performed a *wunder kur* on a neighbor of mine. . . . I know of two cases of similar relief by him, tho' I am unacquainted with the details. It sounds impossible, and I hear that M. is regarded as a quack by medical opinion. Nevertheless, I don't wish to leave that stone unturned, since my own trouble (in which I gladly acknowledge an element of nervous hyperaesthesia) seems progressive. I will let you know the results!" (James). That a man whose opinion we still cherish today should choose a charlatan for himself suggests the continuing need for romanticism in medicine and may explain the popularity of alternative approaches.

To repeat then, as far as I am concerned, many goals of alternative medical practitioners are congenial, but claims that a particular approach has consistent merit must be judged by the same scientific criteria that we use for the placebo or for any other therapeutic agent.

Scientists take data, try to reproduce and categorize them, and then ask why they happen. Alternative practitioners must do the same. I recognize, however, that they will not agree that it is easy to test their approach. They would say that they look for the single best therapy for an individual who has a certain almost idiosyncratic constellation of symptoms and a singular lifestyle and that it would be impossible to fit that patient into a controlled trial.[3]

Mainstream Opinions

Mainstream physicians have much to learn from complementary practices, but I wish that alternative practitioners did not claim so much. Some ideas are right on target, like healing the conceptual split of body and mind in medicine or taking the time to listen to patients, but there remains a collection of theories and practices only a few of which truly offer comprehensive person-oriented care. That makes it difficult to generalize; some alternative practitioners are true believers for whom concepts of health and disease are a religion; their success comes from the dissatisfaction of the American public with the current system. Others are entrepreneurs taking advantage of the holistic health movement to make money.

The attention of mainstream medical practitioners remains directed more to disease than to the person who is sick, and that is a big reason for the growing interest in nontraditional treatments. If 70 to 90 percent of all complaints are now handled outside the usual medical system, the trend early in this century to put all medical care in the hands of licensed medical practitioners has been reversed by the renewed emphasis on self-care.

Mainstream practitioners have looked on alternative approaches as dangerous and ineffective, but they have had to take a second look at the competition. Health maintenance organizations, too, troubled by the "high utilizers" of their product, the members never satisfied by a piecemeal approach, have begun to wonder whether some complementary practices might not only satisfy their clients but also prove cheaper than incessant diagnostic tests. That accounts for some of the growing references to body, mind, and spirit now so popular. As a skeptical Australian, Arthur O'Neill, has suggested, warning about the dangers of alternative medicine implies its effectiveness.

In disdaining placebos and alternative medicine, modern physicians, unlike their postmodern successors, ignore the usefulness of the patient's belief in the therapy and the complementary help of ritual, ceremony, reassurance, and suggestion. They use routine diagnostic tests as placebos even if they do not seem to admit it. That kind of placebo brings reassurance, but I suspect that it is less likely to relieve symptoms than a more positive therapeutic approach does. The postmodern physician who looks at alternatives may be wiser: "If you think it will help, it will."

For many doctors, placebos are "medicine's secret shame," but alternative physicians unabashedly rely on behavioral changes in a way the mainstream disdains. Andrew Weil labels much of what he does as providing "active placebos," in that category including meditation and relaxation techniques and, somewhat less enthusiastically, herbal medicines. All of these implicitly change mind more than body; Bernie Siegel is quoted somewhere as saying that he would give shark cartilage to patients only if it helped their state of mind and gave them hope. Hope is where the action is.

A Partnership

Consideration of placebos, alternative medicine, and other interventions that together treat mind and body could result in a resurgence of psychosomatic medicine. I am heartened by the growing partnership between psychoneuroimmunology, as mainstream as you can get, and alternative medicine. Although their projects begin to look alike, neither seems happy to admit their growing partnership.

As I emphasized in Chapter 1, postmodernism has provided the environment for the reentry of alternative approaches into the mainstream. Postmodernism casts aside the models of modern medicine, but just as the skeleton provides support for the body and makes it possible for us to act on our ideas, without modern science, alternative medicine would be a return to the nineteenth century. I hope that alternative medical ways will clothe the skeleton of biomedicine, so that the real meaning of *complementary* will become clear. Alternative ways may also find a place for the spirit, to bring heart back to the reductionism still so dominant in biomedical theory. Physicians must reawaken to the possibility that more than a few things cannot be measured or imaged, even by medical science, but that this does not lessen their importance.

Nevertheless, problems remain before unification can be complete, and they have to do with language and definitions, as I have already discussed.

One problem stems from the rapid growth of a proactive industry eager to supply the products and pills that alternative practitioners advise. Entrepreneurs are said to be working to convince the Congress that FDA's regulation of dietary supplements has been too stringent, but paradoxically, commercial promotion may bring regulatory controls that may prove more salutary. "Nutriceuticals" have now achieved the attention of industry and bid fair to compete with herbal and other remedies.

Sometimes when I read a claim of alternative medicine or when I have talked with an enthusiast, I find myself wondering what we really have been talking about or what their terms mean. In a very helpful compendium from the National Institutes of Health, from which I have borrowed broadly, many statements in the languages of alternative medicine and biomedicine do not pass the test of translation: can a sentence be translated from one language to another and still make sense?

Neuroimmunologists somewhat prematurely argue that hormones provide pathways for the mind-body dialogue and that stress may wreak its havoc by altering the hormones that modulate immune function. In that scheme, placebos increase hope, which then stimulates hormones or conditioned responses to effect change. The influence of placebos supplements the effect of all drugs because every time we take a pill, hope and expectation—the way of the placebo—enhance its effect.

Medicine is a way of thinking about health and disease, about diagnosis and therapy; modern Western medicine teaches a single mode of perception, and the new impersonal economics, in its latest version of managed care, puts cost ahead of care.

Medical Anthropology

Diseases may be universal, but they are modulated by genetic, environmental, and cultural influences; people in different cultures react to disease and disability in diverse ways, depending on the consensus about an illness and what causes it or what is proper to feel and to discuss. As the ethnic makeup of so many Western countries becomes so diverse, medical anthropology grows in importance. Medical anthropologists study how a culture confronts disease and illness by employing medicines and medical systems. How unpleasant bodily sensations are interpreted will affect what kind of help is sought. Different kinds of practitioners will offer different explanations and find different treatments for the same complaints. Alcohol use offers a common example. Plato's discussion of drinking parties as a "great contribution to education if it is done correctly" would not have gone unchallenged in late nineteenth-century Indiana or in much of late twentieth-century America. In Western society, doctors know that some people with chronic complaints regard them as an expected part of life, whereas others take them as a burden, visiting one doctor after another, searching, usually fruitlessly, for relief.

Studies of medical and folk practices in other cultures also provide a prudent distance from

chapter eleven

Placebos,

Alternative

Medicine,

and

Healing

which to examine Western biochemical models of what it is to be sick. In Western societies being called sick by a physician frees one of responsibilities without stigma, but Western physicians are more ready to accept as sick someone with a disease that can be seen than they are someone with only a complaint, at least until the notion of being "disabled" became generalized over the past few decades.

Robert Hahn illustrates how medical anthropologists think in his book *Sickness and Healing: An Anthropological Perspective*. He expands the postmodern tradition by examining how sickness and healing are conceptualized when the reality of Western medicine is not taken for granted and faults biomedicine for finding science superior to the approaches and methods of non-Western medicines. Unfortunately, as we have seen so often, he conflates illness with disease, using the word *sickness* to mean any "unwanted condition in one's person or self—one's mind, body, soul, or connection to the world," thus defining sickness from the patient's perspective alone. *Healing* becomes the elimination of whatever is unwanted by the sick person in a process "in which social interaction and societal organization play a prominent role, along with the medical or surgical procedures." The patient's story, the narrative, wins the central role in Hahn's version of medical practice. He wants doctors to learn the patient's concepts of disease and their context in the patient's life. His approach substitutes another language for biomedical jargon; and its answers are not always comprehensible to doctors, particularly when he defines healing in nonmedical terms.

The culture-bound syndromes require as much attention as any carcinogen, bacteria, or virus. In proposing an anthropological medicine, Hahn wants doctors to recognize ethnic variability and the importance of accommodating to patient's ideas of why and how they got sick. His notions are especially pertinent to ambulatory practice but less important in hospitals, where character and culture count for much less, and appropriately so, than knowledge and technology.

Hahn defines a placebo as the self-fulfilling prophecy of healing.

Hwa-Byung offers an exotic example of how culture influences the choice of symptoms. The Western clinician who reads of Hwa-Byung among Koreans will recognize a familiar depressive equivalent in the complaints of indigestion, anorexia, dyspnea, palpitation, generalized aches, and a mass in the epigastrium. Upon analysis such patients turn out to be depressed, and in the only English-language report, its psychological origin is underlined.

Among Chinese and Koreans, somatization provides the most acceptable outlet for stress. The Chinese patient with many troubles will not complain, "I am under too much pressure," but only, "I have a headache or a stomachache." Whether the Western metaphor of "pressure" is a better one is a subject all in itself. Chinese medicine is so organ oriented that many Chinese patients are reluctant to express emotions except as somatic complaints. Somatic illness is an "effective and legitimate excuse to request rest and care from others, while psychological strain is not. . . . Thus, patients learn how to present their problems in terms of somatic complaints." So ready an acceptance of somatic illness with so little respect for mental health must make people reluctant to explore their emotional problems. As their culture reinforces hypochondriasis, many Chinese people find bodily sensations a convenient scapegoat.

Practitioners in Taiwan called *tang-ki* treat what Westerners would largely call psychosomatic and emotional disorders: "As we have seen, indigenous practitioners primarily treat three types of disorders: 1) acute, self-limited (naturally remitting) diseases; 2) non-life-threatening, chronic diseases in which management of illness (psychosocial and cultural) problems is a larger component of clinical management than biomedical treatment of the disease; and 3) secondary somatic manifestations (somatization) of minor psychological disorders and interpersonal problems" (Kleinman 1980). Taiwanese patients who go to a Western-style physician for biological diseases choose an indigenous healer for the treatment of fright. Such indigenous therapy may have placebo effects upon such diseases.

Abdominal Pain

We need not turn far for other examples of how culture defines disease. A forty-five-year-old American physician with lower abdominal pain and an unlovable husband may, depending upon her views of life, see a pastor, a lawyer, or any of an array of physician-colleagues. The lawyer may arrange a divorce or a reconciliation; the pastor may strive to keep the marriage together or may act as a therapist, or both. If she chooses a physician, the gastroenterologist, gynecologist, or urologist is ready to invade an orifice to offer an interpretation of what is wrong and give a prescription. Patients from different social classes may give different descriptions of the same sensations. The more sophisticated may talk of stress, whereas the uneducated are still free to talk of pain or "a lizard in the stomach." So often, pain is a cry for help.

A lizard in the stomach figures prominently in Cabot's discussion of lying to patients, and much is made of the bizarre nature of the complaint (see Chapter 9). Lizards, it turns out, can get into the stomach by personalistic or naturalistic routes: "A recurring theme in witchcraft belief is that animals are present in the body, introduced by magical means." In view of Cabot's comments on the woman who complained that she had a lizard in her stomach and in view of the unattributed comments of Freud on this matter, it is interesting to note that animal intrusion as a cause of illness has a long history in European and American folklore. Spring lizards, as well as other animals, grow in the stomach from drinking river water that contains eggs, according to folklore. Fear of having a lizard in the stomach is not, then, quite as unnatural as Cabot apparently believes.

Other physicians might have failed to rout the lizard because they did not possess special powers to keep more from growing; their failure might have had nothing to do with lying about therapy. In some cultures, healing is seen as a gift from God, a gift more important than any training. Where a relatively coherent set of beliefs exists, placebos are no more likely to help than any other agents introduced by an outside practitioner.

A Commentary on Anthropological Studies

Disorders keep pace with cultural changes. In a society without telephones, disturbed people cannot annoy others with phone calls. In a medieval society without clocks, type A behavior must have gone under other guises than an obsessiveness with precise schedules. Anorexia nervosa, a disease of rich and plenty, might go unrecognized in a time of famine or, in the Middle Ages, as in St. Catherine of Sienna, seem to be saintly behavior: the young woman with anorexia nervosa might be seen as heroic because of her fortitude and hyperactivity. In the affluent American society, wrinkles seem a legitimate concern, a disease almost, and face-lifts a triumph of medical skill. The sick-building syndrome could not exist without air-conditioning. Other such examples will come to mind.

Most patients get better because most complaints run their course and fade away, in primitive as well as in civilized life; any intervention may be deemed effective when it comes at the right time to gain credit. Because most illnesses end in recovery, local healers earn credit from their patients and anthropologists alike. When therapy for an illness is sought from both a physician and a traditional healer, the physician may cure the patient, but the healer may get the credit.

Physicians pay little attention to the cultural meaning of disease, but, as I have emphasized, anthropologists fail to distinguish between illness and disease, between complaints and organic processes. Shamans and other alternative medical healers should not be accorded too much credit.

Although modern physicians focus too much on the specific biological cause of diseases and not enough on the economic, social, political, and cultural factors that account for so much human illness, anthropologists too often regard all testimony about clinical improvement as equally acceptable. Anthropologists need more active collaboration with trained physicians to delineate the pain and suffering that can be relieved by the cure of disease.

The following suggests the kind of conclusions that anthropologists enthusiastically reach. "All diseases can be thought of as energy problems . . . they can be detected through pulse diagnosis long before changes are visible microscopically. . . . By the time a disease is developed to a secondary, visible state, it is sometimes already too late to stop it. If a potential disease is caught very early, then precise analysis is not necessary: although the form of a future disease is not yet manifest" (Lock). Controlled trials to establish the accuracy of such assertions about predisease are in order. As I suggest elsewhere, surveillance of healthy people to forestall the later development of disease seems little different, except in rationale.

The distress that is relieved by native healers seems to be from either self-limited disorders or disorders of functional or emotional origin. Even the most respected reports usually describe functional disorders, some of which Western clinicians would see as stemming from depression or hostility or representing withdrawn behavior, and the like, or having to do with pain and suffering, distress, impotence, musculoskeletal disorders, and the like. In a study of rural medicine in Greece, symptoms reported as effects of the evil eye that yield to healers include headaches, dizziness, sleeplessness, weakness, fretfulness, numbness, yawning, and vomiting. These are the same self-limited events or functional diseases that most mainstream physicians would recognize as coming from tension and yielding to any charismatic approach.

Implicit in this discussion is the recognition that physicians must consider depression as a cause of their patients' complaints. Chronic Lyme disease, posttraumatic stress syndrom, and many other current diagnoses will have been ruled out by primary care practitioners, who are unlikely to recognize depression very readily and whose patients are equally unhappy to accept that diagnosis. (This may be changing now that "biologically based brain disease" has replaced "mental illness" in the mind-body spectrum.) Still, many people think of depression as something that they should be able to control by willpower. That is only occasionally true, so in diagnosis the physician must always consider the possibility of depression. As a gastroenterologist, I ask patients, "Does stress, food, or God make your symptoms worse?" The allusion to the Creator is intended as a confession that sometimes we do not know why bad things happen.

Like Robert Hahn, whose teacher he has been, Arthur Kleinman tells us that the biomedical model is not the only one by which medical anthropologists should judge healing. Still, even anthropologists should not equate relief of complaints with cure of disease if there is ever to be mutual understanding across cultures, including science.

Western physicians, nurses, and nurse practitioners, trained to deal with disease in a specific, logical, and rational way, can be open to other forms of therapy without abandoning their logical approach. On the other hand, the faith healer or folk practitioner with no background in rational medicine cannot utilize the scientific approach. Considerations of folk medicine may convince Western practitioners that a number of complaints could be handled outside the usual medical context. There should even be economic incentives to do so, but few doctors or patients recognize that not every complaint deserves a full diagnostic workup.

Psychosomatic Medicine

When doctors call a disease psychosomatic, they mean that it is either caused by or made worse by emotional factors. For the former, psychogenic would be more appropriate, but few diseases fall into that category today. Because most diseases have multiple causes, it is hard to think of a disease whose symptoms do not worsen with emotional stress. Psychosomatic medicine is not a belief that diseases are caused only by the brain/mind. The term should imply that no disease is free of emotional aspects, or—in the terms used in this book— that every disease in every conscious person has an accompanying illness.

Psychosomatic medicine is the study of the interrelations between emotions and bodily processes, either normal or pathological. The implied dualism of mind and body seems unattractive, however, now that we know that such neurotransmitters as cholecystokinin, a hormone found originally in the gut, are also widespread in the brain. Psychosomatic medicine, like many holistic alternatives, sees disease in the context of life. The physician regards the patient as a person and makes no separation of the psychosomatic from the rest of medicine. Psychiatry may have diseases of the mind for its domain, but discoveries during the past decades suggest that mental states have a molecular locus.

Psychosomatic considerations can be traced back to Hippocratic medicine, which was largely somatic, developed to escape the more mystical Aesculapian medicine of the temples. Hippocratic practitioners saw no need to treat the soul or the psyche as such, for they did not distinguish it from the body. Yet Plato remarked on the helpfulness of fair words for the soul, and Galen later directed attention to the role of the emotions in human diseases and hoped to free humans from their passions. Those who think that Norman Cousins had a new idea in healing with laughter should know that Maimonides recommended the stimulation of psychic energies through perfumes, music, and enjoyable stories. In the nineteenth century Connecticut's William Beaumont showed how emotions influenced gastric secretion in his hapless subject Alexis St. Martin.

Holistic postmodern practitioners would have little quarrel with Margaret Mead, who looked at the culture and society of the sick person and noted

> that the functioning of every part of the human body is moulded by the culture within which the individual has been reared. . . . Also by the way that he, born into a society with a definite culture, has been fed and disciplined, fondled and put to sleep, punished and rewarded. In order to understand the pattern of psychodynamics, we had to go to the life history of the individual patient.

> The cultural pattern is built into his whole personality in one process in which no dualism exists so that the temper tantrum, the tautened muscles, the change in the manufacturing of blood sugar, and the verbal insults hurled at an offending parent, all become patterned and integrated.

> The psychosomatic theorist will have made a considerable advance in the invocation of culture in his thinking if he can think of two individuals from different cultural backgrounds, as he might think of the manifestations of Reynaud's disease under different temperature conditions. (Mead)

Those in the psychosomatic movement erred in thinking that a specific personality or a specific way of reacting brought about a specific disease. They foundered on the notion that the psyche causes disease, and could not resolve the mind-brain dilemma. Postmodern physicians accept the mind-brain-body link with enthusiasm, but the idea that the mind-brain worsens diseases but does not cause them persists. Carl Jung's comments encapsulate that old view where he remarks on "a discovery which is very unwelcome to the science of medicine: namely, the discovery that the psyche is an etiological or causal factor in disease. In the course of the nineteenth century medicine shaped its methods and theory in such a way as to become one of the disciplines of natural science, and it also adopted that primary assumption of natural science: material causation."

The naming of neurobiological brain disease attests to postmodern feelings about mental illness. Present-day psychiatrists are trying to regain acceptance as neurobiologists, so they welcome the idea that biochemical or molecular derangements cause mental disorders. Still, the conviction that people are part of their culture and that reactions to specific situations lie embedded in their physiology has been revived as holistic medicine. People are born into a culture; their physiological systems and ways of reacting are as influenced by individual experiences with parents, surroundings, and culture as is language. I like the definition of psychosomaticist as "physician who specializes in listening," like many alternative practitioners.

In the 1930s and 1940s interest in nutrition was almost as avid as it is today, fostered then by the recent discovery of vitamins. Comparing culture to diet has a familiar echo today: "The culture may be likened to the standard diet in which the individual members have subsisted since birth." Those who ascribe changes in gastrointestinal diseases to changes in diet alone, and not to changes in culture, should have some reservations about recommending fundamental changes in the American diet and not in its psyche.

I have related how the suggestion that the FDA permit over-the-counter drugs that are clearly placebos was not taken seriously. A brave psychiatrist in Providence in 1994 proposed that placebos be given to depressed patients, for about a third of moderately depressed patients improve on placebo treatment in controlled trials. He advised that such patients be seen regularly by an interested kind of person who would assess progress, let the patient verbalize distress, and provide practical advice in visits fifteen to thirty minutes long. Patients who did not show substantial improvement after four to six weeks could go on to antidepressants.

That proposal evoked a barrage of comments, most of which dealt with the issue of improvement versus remission, along with comments that the placebo success rate was high only in mildly depressed patients. In wondering whether very brief psychotherapy would do just as well as placebos, the responding psychiatrists seemed to be defending their own usefulness more than the truth of the suggestion.

Personalistic Versus Naturalistic Systems

Systems that have inherently rational bases, however unusual to Westerners, should be distinguished from those that rest on purely supernatural explanations. Social scientists suggest that all healing systems have a rational basis but that sometimes it has been forgotten, leaving a supernatural agency to require actions that once had more obvious reasons. In some societies, religion and medical practice are inseparable; in others, they are as separate as in the West.

Cultures deal with the cause of disease in two ways. In a *personalistic* system, an agent, which may be human, nonhuman, or supernatural, directly causes disease or suffering. In a *naturalistic* system, natural forces or conditions are held responsible; an imbalance of body elements, like the four humors of the Greeks or the yin or yang of the Chinese, can lead to disease. Many contemporary naturalistic systems have hot and cold poles, disease being explained by an excess of one or the other.

Personalistic explanations of disease are part of a worldview, usually religious in origin, whereas naturalistic systems offer an explanation for sickness and nothing more. The two systems have different requirements for a cure. In the first, the shaman, priest, or witch doctor must use magical skills to find out who caused the disease, so that appropriate propitiation may lead to a cure. Achilles, for example, was faced with the plague that was killing the Greek soldiers:

> Rank and file
> sickened and died
> for the ill their chief had done
> in despising a man of prayer.

He asked,

> Why all this anger of the God Apollo?
> Has he some quarrel with us for a failure
> in vows or hekatombs? Would mutton burned
> or smoking goat flesh make him lift the plague?

Naturalistic systems, in contrast, require the more classical doctor who understands the origin of disease and can devise appropriate treatment.

The personalistic approach is less helpful in thinking about placebos; people who believe that they are sick because they have been cursed may respond to placebic intervention, but the personalistic view rises above physiology. Most naturalistic views share the internal logic of a psychosomatic explanation.

Naturalistic systems are more congenial to modern and postmodern physicians, for they explain diseases as arising from an imbalance of principles. Treatment takes a rational, empirical approach, whether through the diets of ancient Greek physicians—or postmodern ones— or the manipulations of the village healer or chiropractor or the needles of the acupuncturist. No matter how primitive, the seemingly logical basis of naturalistic concepts has more in common with modern medical practice than the personalistic tradition, which sees disease as caused by the ill will of an outside agent.

Personalistic Systems
Witchcraft

For most of us, to comprehend witchcraft and what it means to someone raised in a culture with recognized witches requires suppression of a rational approach to medical practice. The wide gulf between science and sorcery was not bridged some years ago when a doctor from Ghana voiced his disappointment that an English psychiatrist missed the spiritual side of the juju houses and fetish shrines of his tribe, taking "demon possession" as only hysterical exhibitionism. Turning to the words of Pascal, "There are two excesses: to exclude reason, to admit nothing but reason," this modern African physician concluded that science has no tools to probe spiritual things that remain suprascientific.

An educated physician like him who accepts the reality of witchcraft looks little different from his religious Western counterparts who accept healing miracles. The witch doctor removing a curse looks very little different, costume aside, from the clergyman casting out a demon or an ancient Greek priest sacrificing hecatombs to Apollo. Similarities aside, empiric evidence or predictability is as much lacking in witchcraft as in faith healing.

Faith Healing

Where you locate the faith that brings healing depends: the secular find it in the recipient and look for responses in immunological apparatus, whereas the religious look for it in the Creator who fashioned those T cells and B cells. Faith healing was defined long ago by Sir Henry Morris, a former president of the Royal College of Surgeons: "In faith healing the suggestion is that cure will be worked by spiritual or divine power, especially if this power be appealed to at some particular place such as a sanctuary, the foot of an idol, a fountain or pool of water. . . . The faith healer does not doubt the reality of matter or of diseases, but believes that he can draw upon a spiritual force to subdue or annihilate an existing evil." Those who claim that prayer and ritual may help seem to praise the utilitarian value of a belief in God, putting more faith in the power of prayer than in the power of the Creator.

The very term *faith healing* is contentious. A friend who is an Anglo-Catholic priest suggests that faith healing puts the locus of healing within the patient or the person who has faith, which is where physicians feel most comfortable putting it, as in hypotheses about placebos. My priestly friend prefers the term *spiritual healing*, for it gives credit to God. His is the personalistic view, whereas most physicians, even religious ones, take the naturalistic one. The conflict is as old as the

Greeks, between the Hippocratic physicians, who believed in science, and the Aesculapians, who helped patients through the mysteries of the temple. My friend may be right, but for now I use the term *faith*, implying that even though God may have created the endorphin system, humans must wake it.

Faith healing in the Christian churches follows from James 5:14–15: "Is any sick among you? Let him call for the Elders of the church; and let them pray over him, anointing him with oil in the name of the Lord: and the prayer of faith shall save the sick, and the Lord shall raise him up and if he has committed sins, they shall be forgiven him."

It is not my purpose to evaluate the miracles reported from time to time, which, curiously, seem to occur in out-of-the-way places, more often in the rural third world than in the urban West. The greatest miracles always seem to occur elsewhere.[1] Morris asked, "How came it about that the Alps and the Pyrenees . . . were so specially selected as the places at which these apparitions and miracles occur?" He explained that the Church did not accept certain miracles of the late nineteenth century "not entirely because France, Italy and Spain are the great Roman Catholic countries of the world, but chiefly, no doubt, for the reason that the inhabitants of the mountain districts are more impressionable to these manifestations."

What to the oncologist is a chemotherapy-induced remission may seem a miracle to the patient, but some sensitive, intelligent, and well-trained physicians believe that true miracles do occur and that fractures can be healed, bleeding stopped, and many other matters beyond scientific explanation can occur as a result of divine grace. I will pass over such events and avoid what Wilfrid Bonser labeled the dangerous field between theology and medicine "that no one has dared thoroughly to explore." I suspect that faith healers, spiritual healers, witch doctors, alternative medical practitioners, and others aim at the same results through the same common pathway. No skepticism is intended, for I believe that healers relieve pain and the emotional component of disease and that the healing touch and transference, the overvaluation of doctors by their patients, are not dissimilar, but I am not equipped to evaluate such claims. After all, healing services are now popular even in Unitarian churches, those bastions of rational thinking.

In *The Wounded Healer*, Henri Nouwen, a Catholic priest, talks of the healing minister: "How does healing take place? Many words, such as care and compassion, understanding and forgiveness, fellowship and community have been used for the healing task. . . . It is healing because it takes away the false illusion that wholeness can be given by one to another. It is healing because it does not take away the loneliness and the pain of another, but invites him to recognize his loneliness in a level where it can be shared. . . . A minister is not a doctor whose primary task is to take away pain. Rather, he deepens the pain to a level where it can be shared."

Faith healing should be a complement, not an alternative to medicine, a collaborative effort that nurtures the *vis medicatrix naturae* within all of us. It seems unlikely that biblical miracles, however, will be rehearsed in our time.

As William Osler describes it, the Emmanuel Movement in early twentieth-century Boston was just that sort of collaboration. This faith healing movement, originated and supported by J. H. Pratt (for whom the Pratt Diagnostic Clinic was later named), offered treatment of nervous troubles by mental and spiritual agencies along with a clergyman and a neurologist.

> Every applicant must first submit to diagnosis. If organic trouble is disclosed, he is not accepted as a patient. If the disease appears to be simply functional, the applicant is registered for treatment and passed on into the Rector's study. There he finds himself in an environment . . . which unlocks the hidden wholesomeness of his inner life and leads by rapid stages to complete recovery. . . .
>
> Where more is needed than the full self-revelation, in itself curative, and the prayer and godly counsel which succeeded, the patient is next invited to be seated in a reclining chair, taught to

relax all his muscles, calmed by soothing words, and in a state of physical relaxation and mental quiet the unwholesome thoughts and the untoward symptoms are dislodged from his consciousness.
(Osler)

This attempt to prevent functional ailments, as well as to cure them, by looking at the whole patient does not sound unfamiliar today.

Christian Science

Christian Science is the most organized of all the religious healing systems. Nathan Talbot of that church wrote, "Disease and physical suffering are in no sense caused or permitted by God, and . . . since they are profoundly alien to His creative purpose, it is wrong to resign oneself to them. . . . Human beings are vastly more than biochemical mechanisms. . . . The basic Christian Science 'diagnosis' of disease involves the conviction that whatever apparent form the disease assumes, it is in the last analysis produced by a radically limited and distorted view of the true spiritual nature and capacities of men and women."

That might seem not too far from a collaboration of care for body and spirit in which placebos might seem the secular equivalent of prayer. Unfortunately for some patients, it is forbidden to combine Christian Science with orthodox medical practice.

Some may think that spiritual healing as practiced by Christian Scientists is acceptable, or at least can do no harm, if employed as an adjunct to medical treatment. The question that then arises is why Christian Scientists believe as they do that their approach to healing cannot successfully be combined with medical treatment. To them this view is not so much a matter of theoretical consistency as one of practical and thoughtful concern for the welfare of patients. As experience shows, the underlying thrusts of specific Christian Science and medical treatment are so dissimilar that to seek healing through both simultaneously is fair to neither of them.
(Talbot)

A patient who turns to medical care is released from the care of Christian Science practitioners "in a supportive spirit and without reproach."

The death of a boy from meningitis while under the care of a Christian Science practitioner led his mother to set up an organization called Children's Health Care Is a Legal Duty. She argued strongly against separating "prayer and support of patients" from the medical care system. In a similar case, when an eleven-year-old boy died from acute complications of diabetic coma, having been treated only by Christian Science prayer and not with insulin, a Minnesota jury ordered the church to pay millions of dollars in damages. A Yale professor subsequently contended that people have a right to educate their children in the religion of their choice. He seemed to ignore the difference between education and medical care; not turning to a physician because of religious beliefs was considered religious abuse by others.

One physician, doubtless impishly, suggested a control trial of Christian Science versus antibiotics for childhood meningitis. He may not have read Peter Medawar's account of Francis Galton's statistical inquiries into the efficacy of prayer. Galton could find no scientific evidence that prayers were answered. In Britain, the queen was prayed for weekly or daily on a national scale, but statistics did not suggest that members of the royal family lived any longer than common people as a result of such prayers on their behalf. Nor could Galton find proof that children of religious parents were less likely to be stillborn than children of the professional classes. Finally, if the devout lived longer than the skeptical, he reasoned that insurance companies would have learned to charge religious believers a higher rate for an annuity because of their longer life. Finding that insurance companies absolutely ignore prayer in making confidential inquiries into the applicant's habits, Galton could not conclude that prayers were answered.[2]

The report to the NIH entitled *Alternative Medicine: Expanding Medical Horizons* has no index list for prayer or Christian Science, although it divides prayer and mental health into two types. In type I, the healer enters into an altered state and merges with the patient; in type II there is a laying on of hands. The author of the executive summary, doubtless wary of treading too far into that demilitarized zone, concludes wisely that it "opens up the power of patients acting on their own behalf"—which would not satisfy my Episcopal friend mentioned earlier but which implies that placebos are the secular equivalent of prayer.

I hope that spiritual healing is not now deemed equivalent to medical care. To read about the ups and downs of the status of Christian Science with legislatures is to realize the power of lobbies and lawyers. Fortunately, as lawyers remind us, religious beliefs, not religious practices, are protected by the Constitution. Anecdotes and narratives alone support the cures of Christian Science—it seems a tragedy that Christian Science prayer cannot be combined with medical and surgical therapy.

Shamanism

Shamans, who used to be called medicine men or witch doctors, have been studied extensively as prototypical spiritual healers. A shaman "uses magic to cure the sick, to divine the hidden, and to control events that affect the welfare of the people"; he or she is a "professional in the field of the supernatural." In reference to the distinction between personalistic and naturalistic medicine, they have been called personalistic specialists who journey by trances to call on the unseen or spirit world to intervene for people in trouble.

If a professional is someone who applies a systematic body of knowledge to problems, the shaman is a professional. If, in addition, a profession must be self-policing and have an abstract body of ideas, shamans look less professional: their methods are empirical but are not subject to the tests of verification and predictability.

Reports of the successes of shamans remind practitioners that many logical schemes can seem to work even though they are flawed from the biomedical standpoint. Most folk medical practices have their own quite different doctrines or methods. Trouble comes when studies comparing shamanistic and biomedical methods of healing consider an "I feel better" from a person whose headache has been relieved by incantation as the equal of the same statement made by someone cured of pneumonia by antibiotics. Conflating subjective reports with objective evidence of healing gives too much credit to the shaman's rate of success. More attention needs to be given to just what it is that shamans help.

Both shamans and modern physicians attempt to establish a logical explanation for any particular illness. "Each uses a specialized approach towards the control of disease, and both approaches are logical. The western physician attacks the problem through an understanding of the parts of the human body machine: its cells, organs, and their functions. The shaman seeks the reason in the supernatural events like the breaking of taboos, magic spells, and the anger of gods" (Rogers).

In the relief of illness, we find many parallels with modern, scientific medicine: "The shaman's first step in attempting to heal is to establish a thorough confidence on the part of the sufferer, his relatives, and other members of the community. They must believe in his supernatural powers and in his ability to deal with the unseen, mysterious forces of health and disease. The shaman draws upon the image of mystic authority that his culture places upon his profession" (Rogers).

Shamanistic methods emphasize the psyche as much as the body: "The shaman's primary attack on the sickness of his patients is psychotherapeutic. . . . Many of his patients, for a variety of reasons, suffer directly or indirectly from emotional disturbance. . . . We can appreciate that his methods, although often bizarre and peculiar to us, can often deal effectively with illness in ways analogous to those used by modern psychiatrists" (Rogers). Psychiatrists might not be so pleased at this analogy. The rest of us might take the shaman as a holistic practitioner who strengthens the bonds of transference, although shamanistic potions may well contain active herbal extracts.

For shamans, disease may be entirely personalistic even though they use holistic methods. The dichotomy between body and mind (or soul), so central in modern Western medicine, has no place in shamanistic therapy. The expectation of being healed is encouraged by dramatic activities that build confidence; most modern physicians, in contrast, feel embarrassed to comfort their patients by their person, using statistics and jargon instead to enforce their authority.

Several features of shamanistic medicine are familiar: relaxation and reassurance, hypnotism, and suggestion; transference and group support. Catharsis brought about by reenactment of the crisis that gave rise to conflict will also have a familiar ring; but symbols and rites give "the patient the feeling that the dread mystery of his illness is being combated by the ancient mysteries of his culture" (Rogers).

Shamans are usually born, not made, and often undergo a wondrous epiphany early in life that gives them a sense of mission; this doubtless contributes to the strength of what can only be called their power of spiritual healing. Michael Harner, an anthropologist turned shaman, tells the fascinating story of how he discovered the way of upper Amazon culture. In his book subtitled *A Guide to Power and Healing* he gave instructions for the shamanic way of healing, which his publisher wisely warned was an adjunct to modern medicine, not an exclusive way of dealing with medical problems.

The shaman is at one pole of the healing process, affecting the mind of the patient. That benefit tells mainstream physicians how much they may be missing out in their cool scientific approach.

Herbal Medicine

In my brief account of shamans I ignored any contribution of the herbs and potions that such healers may use. The lessons of folk medicine and the contributions of native remedies to the pharmacopoeia are well known and are now deservedly under study, but they are not placebos, and have brought a number of untoward side effects along with their benefits.

A Naturalistic System: Chinese Medicine

Chinese medicine, which has developed quite differently from Western medicine, is a mixture of philosophy and empirical science, or tradition. Chinese medicine deals with each symptom as a disease on its own, in terms of the whole body; when the whole is working, there is harmony. What leads to symptoms, called diseases in the Chinese texts, is disharmony, lifestyle, environment, family situations, and much more. Traditional Chinese medicine holds that in health there is a balance between the antipodes of yin and yang. Qi, a kind of energy created by those poles (like magnetism), flows to all parts of the body through channels known as meridians.

Disease results from an excess or deficiency of qi in various parts of the body. Acupuncture needles stimulate these postulated energy pathways, apparent to experts as small spots near the skin surface, to influence the flow of body energy and so restore the healthy yin-yang balance. To identify disharmony and imbalances, the ideal practitioner of Chinese medicine uses many diagnostic techniques, including observation, smell, listening, touch (the twelve pulses), and much more. Important in such diagnoses are colors, dreams, family and social relationships, sexual and physical factors, self-expression, love, spirituality, and recognition that not everything can be explained. The person in pain must be an active agent in rebalancing—not done to by a professional but informed and mobilized throughout. The practitioner, in turn, must see and experience the patient as a whole, not as a collection of symptoms or even imbalances or blockages.

Adepts hold that Chinese medicine focuses on correcting minor imbalances before they become acute; examples of symptoms include low energy, headaches, cold limbs, anxiety, arthritis, nausea from chemotherapy, back pain, painful menstruation, hypertension, and asthma. Such complaints sound very much the same as those that Western practitioners are likely to call functional and treat with tranquilizers or placebos. There are no longer many claims that acupuncture can help such anatomical problems as kidney stones.

Acupuncture for the treatment of drug dependency or addiction has been praised in uncontrolled reports. A number of clinics are treating addicts with needles, but whether the effects depend on the technique or on a close relationship between caretaker and addict remains uncertain.

Most commonly, acupuncture is used to relieve pain by the insertion of needles at set points in the skin, remote from the place where the patient feels the pain. Its reputation was boosted in the West some years ago by reports that it made painless operations possible, but in application it has not lived up to the initial enthusiasm. For abdominal surgery, acupuncture does not bring the needed relaxation of abdominal muscles, nor does it relieve the visceral pain that comes from the stretching of internal organs. In head and neck surgery, nevertheless, abetted by sedatives and narcotics, acupuncture still finds a place.

Acupuncture fits into the system of Chinese medicine, a naturalistic system developed some five thousand years ago to explain and treat health and disease. The Western physician should disregard ancient theories when researching whether acupuncture is effective in a predictable and repetitive manner. Only after determining its routine effectiveness does it make sense to try to find out whether its benefits are more than placebic in origin, for the unusual nature of the procedures in themselves must bring a certain therapeutic effect. No one has ever seen the meridians so important to the theory of acupuncture, but the fervor attending demonstrations of their use evokes comparisons with religious discussions.

Looking on acupuncture as a kind of aspirin for a headache misses "the complex of mind/body causes out of which symptoms derive." As Dianne Connelly has pointed out, "In the West, philosophical traditions and cultures emphasize the concept of 'either/or,' where Eastern traditions emphasize both." Western physicians often, and probably rightly, compare it to placebo intervention, as I have done.

It seems plausible that acupuncture needling raises the level of endogenous opioids in the blood or spinal fluid and that neurohumoral mechanisms should be explored to give acupuncture a Western logical base. So far, there is little convincing evidence in controlled trials that acupuncture relieves chronic pain any better than other techniques or placebos, even though acupuncturists claim effects far more widespread than can be explained by endorphins, gate mechanisms, or the inhibition of pain perception by the large-diameter nerves discussed in Chapter 7. Nor, in the field of gastroenterology, which I know best, are there more than cautionary reports of direct effects on either the function or diseases of the digestive tract.

Modern translations of Chinese medical compendiums leave the Western physician dumbfounded at terms that have no parallels in Western physiology. Meridians are just one example. What are we to make of a discussion of abdominal pain that, among other matters, says, "Stomach rots and ripens food. The Spleen transforms and transposes the refined food essence up to the Lungs" or "the Stomach with its downward movement and the Spleen with its upward movement are like crucial crossroads in the Middle Burner" (Sivin). Nowadays, such terms as the *five phases* have replaced the *five elements*, while terms like the *six warps*, along with *yin* and *yang*, can be seen as attempts to categorize clinical experience and standardize bodily processes so that they can be discussed and classified and a logical scheme constructed.

Traditionally in Chinese medicine there are four broad categories of food that may be bad for the stomach. These include foods too cold, too hot and spicy, too sweet, and too greasy, all of which categories sound very much like those often forbidden by Western physicians. Chinese doctors advise patients not to discuss work while eating nor to return to work too soon after a meal, just the kind of sensible advice that can be heard in any primary care office in the United States.

Research into the mechanisms of acupuncture relief is hobbled by more than a few problems. Acupuncturists and typical research scientists rarely speak the same language even when both speak English or Chinese: most sophisticated researchers know little about acupuncture while most skilled acupuncture experts care little about modern clinical trials, which they reject as unreliable, pointing out that acupuncture therapy depends on individual analysis of patients rather than on a specific diagnosis. Needles are inserted at different rates and angles, depending on the needed balancing. Chinese typically use heavier needles inserted more deeply than Japanese acupuncturists, who may not even puncture the skin. Some use electric currents, and Korean practitioners favor needles only in the hands or only in the ear. Sham acupuncture—applying needles where theory says they should not go, without the patients being aware of the use of "wrong" insertion points—might provide a tolerable placebo control, but at the Office of Alternative Medicine there is considerable disagreement about these points, especially because pain from the needles is essential for analgesia, which makes a control with sham acupuncture—done without the pain of rotating the needles—not a true control.

An assessment of the contending views of acupuncture leads me to

the conclusion that acupuncture relieves pain overall in about 60 percent of patients, a rate not so much different from that with placebos.
The relief of pain by acupuncture is sometimes very quick, almost
immediate, and sometimes slow, and its duration is unpredictable.

Critics are rightly concerned about many of the clinical studies—
claiming relief of chronic pain syndromes, raised endorphin levels, and
even improvement in serious psychiatric difficulties—because of the
absence of control or placebo groups. A leading British homeopathic
physician, George Lewith, agrees that controls using physical placebos
must prove the benefit of acupuncture, but he claims for his own study
only a 30 percent rate of pain relief, which is very similar to placebo
relief rates. George Mendelson, who has conducted controlled trials of
acupuncture, states flatly, "The placebo component is clinically more
important than its physiological effects." One well-designed study of
dysmenorrhea involved sham acupuncture, but the investigator apparently knew who was receiving the sham treatment and who the real.
Moreover, he confessed that the results, which favored real acupuncture, depended, as in so many studies of pain, on statistical manipulations. The abstract of the study report, which is presumably all that
many read, implied much less doubt than the body of the report.

Because there are so many different kinds of experimental and clinical pain and so many different expectations from such different patients, convincing evidence of the mechanism of acupuncture will be
long awaited. How much benefit comes from the person doing the
procedure and how much as a consequence of sustained effort, attention, transference, and hope remains uncertain, a criticism also leveled
at psychotherapy, placebos, and other interventions.

Arguments seem limitless. Chinese physicians retort that many
Western medications have been in use only for a short time and that
their long-term consequences are not clear. Western physicians counter
that Chinese herbal medicines contain extracts that sometimes prove
harmful. Reevaluation of both positions is in order. Postmodern physicians might well agree with a possibly apocryphal Chinese folk practitioner who was heard to remark, "There should be a law that says
people should not start medications for high blood pressure until they

have tried some form of alternative medical treatment." A well-known hypertension expert also has observed that a third of patients with high blood pressure could remain healthy without medication, but surveying them for complications seems so difficult, and their anxiety at getting no medication so great, that he and his colleagues have decided that giving medication is their easiest solution.

Chinese medicine is logical, traditional, holistic, and internally consistent, even if its tenets do not accord with those of Western bio-medicine. Whether it is effective for more than the 80 percent of the complaints that mainstream physicians call illness remains to be seen.

Chinese medicine has kept its philosophical and holistic flair, which might help the Western patients whose aid comes from clergy, psychiatrists, physicians, or just good friends and the healing power of nature. The physiology of Chinese therapeutics is likely to prove faulty, and the good effects of acupuncture may turn out to be placebic in origin, but tradition and mystery help the 80 percent of patients who will be helped by alternative medical practices—or by the passage of time.

There are different ways of conceptualizing the body, but surely an idea lately again popular in the West is not foolish: to consider the body and the person as a united organic entity in balance. There is no word for health in Chinese except for one borrowed from the Japanese. Instead, synonyms like normal, harmonious, and relaxed describe the ideal. "The mind is centered and free from inappropriate immoderate emotions" sounds not very different from the advice of the Greek philosophers. The loose distinctions between diseases and symptoms make evaluation difficult. The authority and success of Western medicine has led to increasing westernization of some of these ideas.

Finally, the Western physician who believes that most of the relief provided by acupuncture comes from perception rather than sensation will be amused at a jingle in Nathan Sivin's book.

> For the belly san-li's for you.
> For the back wei-chung will do.

Head and neck? Look for lieh-chu'u.

Face and mouth? You want ho-ku.

That is not so very different from "An apple a day keeps the doctor away."

Alternative Medicine—Some Other Examples
Biofeedback

Between mainstream and alternative medical practices lies biofeedback. That technique relies on an electric monitor that gives an audible beep or a visible blip on a screen to reflect changes in skin temperature, muscle contractions, blood pressure, or some other physiological function. Spasm of the anal sphincter, for example, brings a quick series of beeps; the patient tries to slow the beeping, and gain relief, by altering breathing, imagining pleasant scenes, or in some other way trying to relax the sphincter. Once that is possible, the sphincter comes under conscious control, so the theory holds; thereafter, the patient should be able to relax the sphincter without biofeedback instrumentation.

There are many different techniques for biofeedback, and they are used by physicians, by alternative practitioners, and even by laypeople on their own. Their value is yet to be assessed.

Homeopathy

Homeopathy has been employed in postmodern times by a number of primary care doctors. Started in the nineteenth century by a German physician, Samuel Hahnemann, as a salubrious reaction to the heroic therapies—like bleeding or purging or cupping—of those times, it later went into decline until brought, in the past ten years, from the backwaters to mainstream influence. Adherents claim that taking a chemical that, when administered, causes the symptoms of a disease and diluting it so much that no molecule remains in the solution, then striking the bottle in which it is contained in certain ways a number of times—a process labeled succussion—imparts healing powers to that medication. The claim that dilution paradoxically makes an agent more powerful has yet to be tested.[3]

Over the past few years several homeopathic preparations have been awarded statistical applause when published in various proud journals.[4] For instance, homeopathic remedies have proven helpful in the management of diarrhea in children in Nicaragua; an editorial lamenting the complexity of the prescribing process failed to credit the accurate and elaborate history taken of mental status, which is certainly an important factor in increasing expectations. That is a major point: homeopathic practitioners see fewer patients per hour than the usual primary care doctors, two to three as against four to five.

We need more discussion of these matters. Homeopathy may bring benefits, as do so many other alternative forms of medicine, because its practitioners are friendly and unhurried, taking into account the patient's values and teaching that illness is part of life, to be overcome when it cannot be eliminated.

Chiropractic Medicine

Chiropractic medicine has a very long history and is licensed in every state in the Union, as well as in many other countries. Because it now has forty-five thousand practitioners in the United States alone, it should not be considered alternative medicine, but because the NIH manual on the topic includes it, I summarize its position here.

Chiropractors are concerned with the relation between structure of the spine and function of the human body. In the belief that the body has an innate self-healing ability and that the nervous system influences all other bodily systems, chiropractors consider that joint dysfunctions and what are termed subluxations, a kind of dislocation, interfere with the normal action of the neuromuscular system. For that reason, chiropractic physicians use hands-on techniques to make diagnoses; their treatments for various problems largely involve manual manipulations. By law, they may not employ surgical or chemotherapeutic approaches.

Reading about the history of chiropractic medicine and its many schisms and founders, a skeptic might well find a parallel with religious history. In general, patients with back pain and neuromuscular problems have been helped by manipulations, but the jury is still out for other complaints. In a 1991 judgment (*Wilk et al. v. The American Medical Association*) it was held that mainstream medical groups had restrained trade by restricting consultation between chiropractors and mainstream doctors, but chiropractic medicine has a long way to go in setting standards for procedures and review. Still, a 1995 report of the outcome of treatment for low back pain found that patients were more satisfied with chiropractic treatment than with treatment from primary care doctors. Sadly, other reports find just the opposite: that chiropractic is not better than standard treatment. As the phrase goes, more studies are needed.

Dance Therapy

Among the techniques of mind-body therapy is dance. Dance is, after all, one way the body gives its emotions visible reality, so the analogy with medical practice, which searches for meanings in that too often silent body, is not without foundation. Visible movement expresses personality, as doctors who recognize depression by bodily clues already know. Dance is an almost universal way to celebrate joy, so no one should be surprised that it has been used in healing rituals. Comparisons between hysteria and dance have been noted as well. Dance therapy aims at helping people with social, emotional, or similar problems express their feelings.

Music Therapy

Music, too, has roots in human history, with "charms to soothe a savage breast." Music engages the emotions directly, without the delay of intellectual processing; it has power to cheer up people, including patients. If positive emotions benefit healing, physicians might consider enlisting music therapy to lift the spirits of the depressed or to help those in chronic pain, paralyzed patients with emotional problems, or even people with dementia. Other appeals to the creative and emotional side of human nature at first glance seem wide of medical practice, but questions shake our certainty. Can the person with Alzheimer's disease be recalled a little by familiar music or familiar odors?

Does that do any good? Such questions, which cannot be answered here, show how far complementary approaches have gone.

We will not soon be certain how much the brain, whether mind or neurons, influences the body. Nor is it now possible to dissect out the specific virtues of alternative medicine beyond its mobilization of attention and perception. Still, a study of hypertension in Sweden a few years ago showed that young men in high stress occupations had higher blood pressure at work than others did, and the same is true of blacks in the still biased American society. Stress and strain elevate blood pressure by activating the sympathetic nervous system, so it is not surprising that relaxation therapy and similar approaches have reduced blood pressure. The therapy might have been nonspecific and even placebic, for Harvard researchers have concluded that cognitive therapy reduces hypertension only in so far as it is a credible placebo. Alternative medicine practitioners do need to ask research questions even if they are content only to help. The brain does speak to the body's organs.[5]

Although physicians once used placebos frequently, now they usually deny ever giving them, as if to do so would be putting something over on patients. On the other hand, they often prescribe impure placebos, probably to keep from recognizing what they are doing. As we have seen, this new guilt at using placebos has its origin in the biomedical mode, based on physics, which takes the body for a machine and the brain for its computer. Fear of playing the charlatan also has a part. Yet if placebos are effective, doctors must admit that their scientific models do not explain everything. Allegiance to science defines the profession, but it need not limit what doctors can do.[1]

Training Physicians: Reason Versus Intuition

The scientific, rational basis of modern medicine conflicts with its priestly mystical heritage. Mainstream Western physicians try to analyze logically and base their treatments on reproducible phenomena. Diagnosis—in internal medicine, if not in dermatology—depends on being able to predict what you will see from what you hear from the patient, and prognosis depends on confidence that what has happened before will happen again. The contrast between *reason*, which measures, and *intuition*, which grasps in a flash, goes back to the Greeks and even to ancient Egypt, where attempts to measure physiological behavior were common in Alexandria in the third century B.C.

Hippocratic medicine was the rational side of medicine, characterized by knowledge of natural sciences, practical experience, reasoning about cause and effect, and ethical concepts. In contrast,

chapter twelve

Why

Doctors

Don't

Like

Placebos

priestly or Aesculapian medicine relied on dreams, oracles, and miracles and the caprices of the gods and lacked any consistent sequence of cause and effect. Hippocratic physicians were empiricists who distrusted revealed dogma as much as modern doctors do. Nor did they trust their patients much more, regarding what they had to say as mere opinion. For such reasons, Lain Entralgo tells us, Virgil called medicine the silent art.

The followers of Aesculapius, whose staff, entwined with a single serpent, has remained the symbol of modern medicine, built temples near the sea and adorned them with works of art—there is a resemblance here to many modern American hospitals looking for customers. Baths, abstinence, and ceremonies, interpretation of dreams, and even hypnotic states all formed part of the cure. The healing scene must have been as impressive as at the referral centers of today; ceremonies strengthened the faith that patients brought with them and surely helped cure complaints that we would now call illness. Even the rational and empirical Greek physicians were influenced by religious ideas: "When the art of the physician fails, everybody resorts to incantation and prayers." The same is true today.

At Ephesus, Turkey, where Artemis had been worshiped and where St. Paul preached against cults, a large medical center has been excavated. The patients drank herbal potions to make them sleepy, and as they walked down the long underground passage, the priests whispered words of healing suggestion, pretending these came from the gods.

The Iliad offers a striking contrast between diseases brought on by the whimsicality of the gods, which could be cured only by priests sacrificing animals, and battle wounds, which could be treated by laymen but which were better treated by physicians. For plagues brought on by the gods, sacrifices and other forms of propitiation were deemed more effective than the logical approaches of physicians. To a great extent, physicians in the Iliad work largely as trauma surgeons, dressing wounds, staunching blood, and relieving pain.

Two Kinds of Knowledge

In ancient Greece, knowledge was of two kinds, measuring and nonmeasuring; even so, classification and description were more important than measurement.

In the Middle Ages the seven liberal arts were divided into the trivium (grammar, rhetoric, and logic), which had to do with verbal methods of analysis, and the quadrivium (arithmetic, geometry, astronomy, and music), which dealt with measurement and calculation. Later, as faith waned and the sciences rose in general estimation, the trivium yielded to the quadrivium, leaving our word trivial as a hint of the low regard for that first group. Yet a noted medical historian, Lina White, exhorts:

> What must be denied is that mathematics, measurement, and quantification provide much insight into the deepest personal problems and experiences of our race: courage and cowardice, affection and hatred, generosity and greed, charm and repulsion, courtesy and boorishness, awe and mockery. . . . About such matters we can only talk to each other . . . not expecting to arrive at 'laws' but rather at rough consensus that draws on long experience and take a long view of the road ahead. Quadrivial ways are useful, but those who employ them habitually because they produce good harvest from their special fields must recognize more vividly the severe limitations of their favorite method. (White)

The emphasis on quantification arose during that remarkable period in the eighteenth century called the Enlightenment, which brought faith that scientific techniques can give rational answers to all problems. The scientific method had already achieved such triumphs in the world of physics that it seemed likely to do the same in all fields of human endeavor—social, literary, and spiritual among them. Isaiah Berlin has described the central principles of the Enlightenment as "universality, objectivity, rationality, and the capacity to provide permanent solutions to all genuine problems of life" (Berlin). It follows that "the Enlightenment adopted mathematics as the science of sciences."

The Counterenlightenment came along as a reaction to this rational, logical approach and its claims of universality; it culminated in the romantic movement of the nineteenth century, "with its faith in the authority of revelation, sacred writings and other non-rational and transcendent sources of knowledge." For some in the Counterenlightenment, faith in God, religious experience, and the inner life of each individual seemed more important than any truth brought by the senses.

In the early eighteenth century Giovanni Vico of Naples proposed that there were cycles in cultural development, not the ever advancing spiral that modern scientists imagine. Each culture is unique, its questions and answers in no way comparable to those of another culture; symbols mean different things at different times to different people. Vico sounds like the best candidate for the patron saint of medical anthropology and for postmodern diversity. Medical practices have to be understood in terms of their own structure and cultural heritage.

The romantic movement was a reaction to the sway of rationality, but unaccountably it had little influence on mainstream medical practice, which has continued to rely on hard data. That accounts for the firewall between alternative and mainstream practices until our postmodern period, with its return to homeopathy, acupuncture, and other alternative approaches.

Science or Intuition?

The contest between reductionists in the medical mainstream and alternative medicine practitioners has its origin in these earlier intellectual currents. The Enlightenment valued only rational thought, but later the Counterenlightenment tried to balance reason with mysticism. Whether we look at folk medicine anew or trace medical practice from the antipodes of Hippocrates and Aesculapius we find the same alternatives. Western medical practice has alternated between these poles of reason and intuition, and the postmodern period represents the latest of those swings. Doubtless some observations have been wrenched to fit my prejudices in what follows, but the lens of the placebo has helped me to focus on these two poles.

Reductionists have no room for complementary views, for they see men and women as their bodies, with organs that can be measured, imaged, and replaced. Education in science makes most doctors view the history of medical practice as a mighty climb away from intuition and romanticism toward reason and logic. Teachers in modern medical schools want to be acclaimed as scientists, and very few are content to be poets. Until the twentieth century, the intellectual climate played a role in medical thought because physicians, among the educated few, were more active in intellectual life in the past than they are today, when medical education is quite separate from the intellectual climate of the wider world.

In some ways medical theory at the end of the twentieth century looks like a fossil unchanged since the scientific revolution. Mainstream medicine has little room for romanticism or intuition and enshrines the rational approach of the Enlightenment. Psychiatrists once examined the emotional background of men and women, but many psychiatrists are so anxious to prove themselves logical scientists that in their studies they have replaced the mind with the brain. Neurobiology holds sway in most psychiatric departments where the fifteen-minute session to adjust medications has replaced the fifty-minute hour to consider the patient's dreams. Psychopharmacology has achieved wonders in the management of depression, schizophrenia, and other brain diseases, but it has not yet located love or ambition or pride or any of the other passions. Freud was, after all, a romantic who thought mistakenly of himself as a scientist. The holistic alternative medicine movement represents the romantic reaction to the sway of reason in medicine in our postmodern time.

We humans live in the two worlds of body and mind. To many, the mind seems much more than our brain, but it would be as foolhardy to praise alternative medicine for treating mainly the mind as it would be to emphasize the logic of rational medicine in focusing on the body. There is a place for mind and brain, for both neurobiology and psychiatry. The Counterenlightenment and romanticism tell us again and again that physicians must recognize men and women as more than collections of organs, as people with plans and hopes, each unique, with strivings and purposes, with deep feelings and intuitions. Fortunately, postmodern practices are letting that idea drift back into the main-stream.

Medical Education in the United States

A major font of resistance to romanticism comes through the train-ing of physicians, standardized for the United States by the famed Flexner Report of 1910. Surveying American medical schools at a time when there were many "uneducated and ill-trained medical prac-titioners," Abraham Flexner found a tide of "unprepared youth . . . drawn out of industrial occupations into the study of medicine" for the sake of profit. The reader today is left to ponder whether medical students at the end of the century are any different from those at its beginning.

Though hired to provide a disinterested view of medical education, Flexner predictably supported the forces promoting science, in Europe as well as in the United States. He silenced consideration of what could not be measured and reduced to facts; he confined the currents of practice to the mainstream, damming up any alternative approaches.

In contrast to present enthusiasm for doctors to become family practitioners, Flexner did not want to train two kinds of physicians, scientists for research and practitioners for family doctors. He believed that bedside practice required a working hypothesis fully as much as laboratory investigation. "The practitioner deals with facts of two categories. Chemistry, physics, biology enable him to apprehend one set; he needs a different apperceptive and appreciative apparatus to deal with the other, more subtle elements. Specific preparation is in this direction much more difficult; one must rely for the requisite insight and sympathy on a varied and enlarging cultural experience. It goes without saying that this type of doctor is first of all an educated man" (Flexner). Flexner wanted to clear away the many nonscientific medical schools and other sources of healing. Ten years later, most of them had closed, leaving the ideal of the physician as scientist.

A child of the Enlightenment, Flexner had no tolerance for what was not scientific. Modern scientists admit that theory often decides which facts they select, but medical educators and physicians mainly look at matters the other way around. Flexner wrote that medical sects needed "theories only as convenient summaries in which a number of ascertained facts may be used tentatively to define a course of action." Theory followed facts in the scientific mode but preceded them in the empirical mode. Not many philosophers of science would agree with him today, but the notion that a theory is built on the painstaking acquisition of facts or observations is still congenial to his medical heirs today, who believe that facts come faster than the theories to explain them.

Emphasizing science in medical school brought together two contradictory goals. Training doctors for practice and expanding medical knowledge are not always well done by the same people or even at the same institution. Training practitioners was the responsibility of hospitals and clinics, whereas expanding scientific knowledge remained the province of universities. The changes that managed care has brought about—for instance, by selling university hospitals to profit-making medical chains—may encourage a return to the British model; there basic scientists work in university departments while clinicians practice in teaching hospitals, imparting their craft to medical students.

Two Hurdles: Science and Residency

The resistance of modern physicians to placebos comes in part from what Berlin has called the scientific fallacy—the faith that all matters can be solved by quantitation. *Reductionists* is the modern term for the same people that William James called medico-materialists. Medical practice is not alone in embracing the scientific fallacy; anthropologists, sociologists, psychologists, and members of most other learned professions have accepted the idea that the techniques of the hard sciences will give permanent answers, that assigning or creating a number makes the answer scientific. The objectivist tradition had three basic assumptions then as today: (1) every genuine question has one true answer; (2) a rational, logical method will lead to correct solutions; and (3) there are universal, eternal, and immutable laws. That was, Berlin emphasizes, "the hour of the greatest triumph of the natural sciences." Goethe somewhere warned, however, that although measurement was useful in the strictly physical sciences, biological, psychological, and social phenomena would elude quantitation and abstraction. The ways of the scientist triumphed as philosophers agreed that logic and rationality could give all the right answers.

Ludwig Wittgenstein neatly summarizes the scientific fallacy. "Our craving for generality has another main source: Our preoccupation with the method of science. I mean the method of reducing the explanation of natural phenomena to the smallest possible number of primitive natural laws; and, in mathematics, of unifying the treatment of different topics by using a generalization. Philosophers constantly see the method of science before their eyes, and are irresistibly tempted to ask and answer questions in the way science does."

This scientific fallacy has been responsible for two major hurdles of medicine that persist today. The first is the hurdle of science. To matriculate at a medical school, the would-be physician must do very well in organic chemistry, physics, and other scientific disciplines. In later professional life doctors may never use that knowledge, but students must evince a fundamental loyalty to science. In addition, passing a course in organic chemistry is said to display the energy and the stamina of the student who would be a physician.

The second hurdle is the hospital-based residency, which has become so very technical that it bears little relation to what most practitioners do. Physicians and educators must ask themselves whether these two hurdles are still as relevant as they once were.

Physicians thus live in two worlds: the world of science, which provides them with their knowledge of disease, very real advances against those diseases, and current ideals, and the world of people, with instincts, pain, suffering, hope, and joy. The first is the universe of physics, the second the realm of the poet. For a long time medicine was first an art and only second a science. That world of the physicist, however, has provided the most attractions for physicians who look on the humanities as providing refreshment but little education. They have embraced the scientific fallacy.

In looking to molecular biology for the answers to pain and suffering, doctors mistake a part for the whole. To avoid any taint of charlatanry, they avoid anything that smacks of intuition. Clinicians used to attend to their patients and leave the function of organs to pathologists or biochemists, but now they, too, prefer smaller units.

That is easy to understand. Physicians treat persons in whom personal, social, and psychological components influence manifestations of disease. Looking around, they do not find great advances in the understanding of "man" or "society." When they study disease processes in which quantification has been responsible for major advances, they conclude that scientific methods offer the only triumphs. Physicians nowadays know so much more about lupus than about lust that they cannot be blamed for believing that quantification should yield answers even to desire.

Clinicians no longer ask why physics rather than poetry should hold their attention, so exciting have been the discoveries of painstaking measurement. For physicians, the scientific method has given the quietus to anything that relies on intuition, mysticism, or irrationality. Repression, as Franz Alexander puts it, is their defense: "Medicine, this newcomer among the exact sciences, has the typical mentality of all newcomers. It tries to make one forget its dark, magical past and therefore it has to watch out carefully that nothing suspicious should remain in it which could betray these undesirable remnants of its prescientific period. Physics, this aristocrat of the natural sciences, can better afford to overthrow its basic principles and undergo a profound reorientation, whereas medicine feels it necessary to emphasize its exact nature in keeping out of its field everything that seems to endanger its scientific appearance" (Alexander 1933).

Modern physicians do not want to be considered charlatans. As the word is defined in the Oxford English Dictionary, charlatan means "an empiric who pretends to possess secrets esp. in the healing art; an empiric or imposter in medicine, a quack." Charlatans claim hidden or mysterious powers arising from their person or from arcane knowledge. Scientists claim only what has been observed and measured, developing hypotheses to explain observations and then testing the hypotheses.

The charlatan does not test experience nor change hypotheses when observations contradict them.[2]

Science sometimes provides a ritual by which physicians keep uncertainty at a distance; laboratory reports to two or three decimal points give a specious aura of accuracy to medical practice. Working in a research laboratory during training accustoms young physicians to believe that precise measurements bring certainty. Most men and women enter clinical practice, but they keep that training for precision in their hearts.

Medical students and even practicing physicians are often in despair at all the facts and numbers they are supposed to keep in their heads, and are happy to turn them over to computers. Most go to medical school to learn to take care of patients, but then they find that medical practice is focused on numbers.

Physicians have largely forgotten their place in the world of people and have an eye only for diseases, their vision blinded by science. Scientists stand at the frontiers of the unknown, looking ahead; technicians look backward to measure what is predictable. Medical research in the course of clinical training sometimes passes only that technology test. Scientists find phenomena that challenge current theories, then say, "Well, I don't know why this should happen. According to our theories, it doesn't make sense, but here it is! Therefore, let's look into the matter, revise our theories and figure out why."

Indeed, some time ago in the *New England Journal of Medicine* the model of physician as engineer was praised. "People need to be understood as causal systems very much as do bridges and boats and airplanes and bacteria. Without understanding people as objects in this way, there can be no such thing as medical science."

The Objectivity of Facts and Observations

Physicians forget how theory-driven fact-finding is. Even in the hard sciences, there is increasing awareness of the perceptual baggage that the scientists bring with them and the way culture and preconceptions determine what we see and study. For example, many lawyers have no very solid notion of law as discoverable; rather, they recognize that law is created, determined by culture and society. Philosophers will no doubt always try to arrive at a universal ethic, but pragmatists argue that culture determines what is, temporarily, ethical. Science is no different.

Wittengenstein emphasizes how much seeing is really "seeing as." Looking at an ulcer crater, I see a white spot with depth and a little edge of redness, but I immediately see it as an ulcer crater because of my experience. The subjectivity of such an approach is evident. In this regard, "Nature imitates art," said Oscar Wilde, in three words encapsulating a theory. The artist gives us a new reality: we accept the artist's view, at least temporarily. A preindustrial man before a word processor would see its keys but could not put them into a context, would not really know what he or she saw. There is so much to find in this universe of ours that scientists would be lost without some preconceptions. As Peter Medawar puts it, "We cannot browse over the field of nature like cows at pasture." Or, as Albert Einstein told Werner Heisenberg, "On principle, it is quite wrong to try founding a theory on observable magnitudes alone. In reality the very opposite happens. It is the theory which decides what we can observe" (Heisenberg).

Even physicians trained as scientists cannot avoid looking at alternative approaches if only because the laypeople who are their patients are so intrigued by them. Even though they may not doubt the sufficiency of the scientific approach, physicians must pay more attention to the nonrational forces in human nature, which the arts and the humanities, psychiatry and psychoanalysis, help us begin to understand.

Ethnic or Cultural Medicine

The notion that there might be a culturally based social or ethnic medicine specifically Chinese or Greek or African used to seem farfetched. Because enzymes, genes, and cells function in human bodies much the same way around the world, ideas that ethnic, cultural, or emotional differences play a role in the response to disease still seems to many physicians a temporary superstition that the triumphs of science will eliminate.

Yet cultural patterns influence how medicine is practiced. Japanese doctors in Japan view therapy for dying patients quite differently from the way their Japanese American counterparts do. Japanese doctors are not likely to tell patients that they are dying, and they recommend blood transfusions and other life-supporting measures for patients whom American-born physicians of Japanese ancestry would not treat. Heart transplants have not been done in Japan since 1968, and abortions are very common. The average length of stay in a hospital in Japan in 1990 was almost forty-five days, far longer than the week or so average stay in an American hospital, whether for what an American physician might consider unnecessary treatment or in the best interests of the patient. These differences are rooted not in science but in culture.

Look at how physicians now study the patient whose dyspepsia resists treatment, trying antibiotics, doubling the dose of acid-blocking agents, endoscoping the patient over and over again, talking of an operation and running statistical trials. Yet none of those explain the 10–15 percent of ulcer patients who do not respond to therapy or who suffer an endoscopic recurrence without any symptoms. Ulcers may recur, but physicians, astonishingly, ignore psychological features that may contribute to that recurrence. The ulcer is their target, along with smoking and other bad habits of patients, but the fears or stresses of the person who has the ulcer are ignored.

Induction and Deduction

The difference between charlatanry and science mostly comes down to the difference between induction and deduction. Induction is arguing from the particular to the general, whereas deduction is arguing from the general to the particular. As Medawar so nicely puts it, "Inductivism in scientific papers [is] simply the postures we choose to be seen in when the curtain goes up and the public sees us." Induction is the development of a theory from a set of facts, but, as Medawar knows, "scientists select out facts to build their theories or probably more properly to buttress them." Physicians are trained in induction; the primacy of facts and observations has gone unchallenged, even though many scientists have talked of intuition bringing an idea unbidden, sudden and entire. Medicine is no different. That medical practice is more than molecular biology, that humans are more than collections of chemicals, still appeals to many postmodern physicians who hope that thought is not reducible to brain events.

The scientific method does not mislead, but it need not be the only source of inspiration for physicians. In pointing out the dogmatic character of science, Paul Feyerabend, a polemical philosopher, has noted that few question the scientific method because all are indoctrinated in it. People decide whether their children will be taught religion but not whether they will be taught physics or astronomy. Science is one way to understand nature, but the idea that there is no knowledge outside science, he warns, is a fairy tale: "A science that insists on possessing the only correct method and the only acceptable results is ideology."

Scientific chauvinism has no place in a profession that deals with people much more than with diseases. As Feyerabend puts it, "Voodoo has a firm though still not sufficiently understood material basis, and a study of its manifestations can be used to enrich, and perhaps even to revise, our knowledge of physiology." Some hypotheses deserve testing before others, some can be ignored, but we should not ignore myths, dreams, and like experiences. In this regard, Carl Jung makes the point that "if, for instance, a general belief existed that the river Rhine had at one time flooded backwards from its mouth to its source, then this belief would in itself be a fact."

What Can Be Done?

Medical education has long emphasized the scientific measuring aspects of knowledge, ignoring the social sciences, like anthropology and sociology. Medical metaphors may change, but they are always active: the physician procures information, discovers facts, fights disease. Medical practice has followed the objectivist idea. Psychiatry bloomed during the late nineteenth and twentieth centuries, uncovering dimensions to our mental side; but now even psychiatrists have become reductionists, thanks to the victories of serotonin re-uptake inhibitors.

The trouble is that physicians have no very clear concept of what they mean by *human* or *life* or, more important, *death*. It is too bad that they don't discuss such topics as disease, illness, health, pain, and patients; they could talk about whether disease is an entity or whether what counts is how the person with the disease feels and reacts. Lawyers and judges and ethicists can tell them when someone on life support systems is dead, but physicians ought to talk more about what it means to live or die.

In discussions of whom to keep alive, who deserves scarce resources, and more, all of us need to agree on what we mean by a person. In discussing abortion, we do not even agree on what to call the contents of the uterus. Proponents of abortion talk of the fetus even just before term, whereas their foes refer to the unborn child from conception on. These important definitions are fraught with religious concerns, but physicians need to deepen their own definitions by continuing to discuss and read.

Physicians often tell me that soft arguments are of little interest to them: How little different is our understanding of human nature today than it was one hundred years ago? If a twenty-year period can move us from helplessness in treating heart disease to the miracles of heart surgery, then surely such victories are the forerunner of what science will someday teach us about character. But people cannot be yanked whole and entire into the world of science. That many doctors think they can, just because people's organs and diseases can, is attributable to their standard education.

I sometimes compare scientific education in medicine to training tailors by having them study polyester chemistry. They study the molecular structure of wool to learn how sheep raised in different climates produce different kinds of wool. Later they study how cotton grows, when to pick it, and how its fibers are twisted into yarn. They work in a factory for a year making cloth and then, after mastering all the fundamentals, they go out and make clothes. When will they learn to make a suit? They will learn by doing! But such a tailor might not sew a very fine seam.

Clinicians and medical educators have little enthusiasm for comparing physicians to tailors, for there is much more to medicine than technology; still, the analogy to medical education may not be so far off.

After medical school, doctors train for three or more years in hospitals taking care of the very sick. Although training for what will largely be an office or ambulatory practice, they spend much of their time dealing with the high technology of hospitals and learning to divide patients into collections of diseases they can treat. That was fine forty years ago, when practicing physicians cared for sick patients in the neighborhood hospital. Now, however, interns become enormously skilled at activities that will form a very small part of their later tasks and, indeed, are soon outdated in any case. A chief of cardiology once remarked to me how glad he was to spend a month as the attending physician in the coronary care unit because that way he got the chance, once or twice a year, to catch up on what was new. A resident in internal medicine told me how nervous she was about going back to that same coronary care unit because "now they unload the left ventricle, and I don't know how to do that!" The technology of medicine moves on so very fast that what is cutting-edge one year is old hat the next.

Now there are specialists in emergency care, and soon there even may be "hospitalists" to treat the acutely ill patients in our hospitals, which have become large intensive care units. Medical education does not yet prepare physicians for dealing with patients in pain or with chronic diseases. In primitive cultures, religion and medical practice may be one. But Feyerabend was right: for most physicians science has become religion.

The scientific approach has been the origin of much that is worthwhile in medicine. Yet just as mental events soar above brain events, so, too, the informed imagination plays a role in human life, and in human illness. Even if the triumphs of placebos are largely symbolic, that is still a victory. We all live in two worlds: that of scientific achievement, where drugs cure pneumonia, but also in that other more mythical place where comforting words have power over sorrow.

More attention to that second world is needed. Medical students should study science and logic and maybe even mathematics to become expert in rational medicine; but history, fiction, and poetry will teach them something of the "trivial" other side. Discussion of the humanities in medical school and in practice will not detract from their data base, but it will help physicians to respect emotional and social issues, reminding them that humans are more than their biology and that medical practice is more than molecular events.

The American Board of Internal Medicine lists the humanistic qualities of physicians as integrity, respect, and compassion. *Integrity* is defined as "the personal commitment to be honest and trustworthy," *respect* as "the personal commitment to honor others' choices and rights," and *compassion* as "an appreciation of suffering and illness without excessive emotional involvement."

I would add loyalty and empathy to that list.

Placebos work. *The major question* is how. Placebos
may provide an illusion: People go to doctors
when their symptoms are at their worst and after
they have stood them as long as they can. Because
most complaints go away on their own, placebos
or alternative medicine or something else gets
credit for natural history.[1] Alternative practices are
preferable to placebos because they awaken self-
help and self-healing; they are no illusion, for they
encourage activity, not passivity. What follows refers largely to placebos, whose mechanisms have
been studied by mainstream researchers.

Relief of Pain and Suffering

By now it must be clear that I am convinced
that placebos relieve pain and suffering—and no
more—in many different ways, of which changed
perception is paramount. The power of the imagination, Montaigne long ago suggested, can make
us well or sick, or—I would add—make us feel
that way. Most experimental studies dealing with
pain and its relief find that the mechanisms are
psychological, even when endorphins are involved. Miracle cures turn phantasmagoric under
scrutiny; a few commentators tell of dramatic
cures, but in their explanations they return to
brain events. In examining the potential mechanisms by which pain and suffering are relieved, I
will consider only changes that follow shortly after
a placebo is given, for it is hard to assess physical
changes that much later seem to follow a change
in an earlier mental state.

Placebos can bring benefit even when the physician intends to deceive, but only when the patient has faith. This shows the power of hope and

faith, even if respect for truth and concern for informed patients no longer allow most physicians to use placebos in that way. Placebos help even when used as a challenge, and that deepens their mystery.

Animal Studies

It is hard to study the placebo response in animals because we have no way of knowing what a dog feels when it wags its tail, salivates, or modulates its immune responses. My wife's dog is easygoing and noncompetitive. When she swims after a tennis ball, she looks to either side to see if other dogs are also racing for it; if so, she turns tail and leaves the chase. I have no more right to assess her emotional state than other observers have to decide what their animal subjects feel.

Conditioned behavioral responses are studied in animals and, by implication, in humans. Conditioning modifies immune responses in rats, which makes it easier to imagine that receiving pills from a physician may activate responses conditioned in the infant by loving relatives. Animal experiments suggest part of what happens in humans, but people are much more than their behavioral responses.

Anyone, patient or subject, who has ever been relieved by analgesics will have a placebo response stronger than someone who has had little to do with doctors. Such conditioning can be associated with a white coat, a hypodermic needle, entrance into the doctor's office or even just the phone call making an appointment. To the extent that doctors and their therapy have previously brought relief, a patient's response will be favorable, but the opposite is equally true. Placebos can be overdone: patients who get them repeatedly find less and less relief, because the conditioning stimulus grows weaker.

The Mind-Brain Apparatus

As we have seen, a major problem with placebo relief of pain has to do with whether the pain was going away anyway. The mind-brain dichotomy figures strongly in most explanations, but the domains of psychiatry, which studies the mind, and neurobiology, which studies the brain, are a long way from confederation. Those who hold to the brain as a machine-computer focus on mechanisms discussed in Chapter 7. They consider all mental disease or mental effects molecular in origin: depression is a derangement of serotonin metabolism, or perhaps hard-wired neural connections sprouted during fetal life and childhood in a way that makes the early environment responsible for later behavior. Those to whom the mind adds up to more than the sum of its fixed structural components look to ideas or symbols that stimulate the placebo response, and talk about conditioning. No one has yet subjected the brain of someone taking a placebo to positron-emission tomography (PET) scans or to magnetic resonance imaging to watch what happens in the brain. Most explanations of placebo responses remain conjectural.

Behavioral Mechanisms

Why some people respond to placebos and others do not remains a mystery if everyone has the same biological apparatus. That a third of us are very good placebo responders may be traced genetically, like color-blindness or, as I believe, to specific learned ways of responding to certain stimuli. Like being a good basketball player, you have to practice.

There are two types of theories: (1) mental, having to do with thoughts, and (2) conditioning, having to do with changes in observable behavior. Mental theories take into account hope, anticipation, and other constructive emotions that are beyond current display on video monitors but that have to do with perception. Conditioning encompasses stimulus-response and learned behavior. Even if the placebo response proves largely mental, its benefits deserve respect. The public likes to read about how alternative practices stimulate natural healing processes, but these mysteries are difficult to define beyond the tendency of any healthy body to repair itself. We should remember that healing has a different meaning for most doctors than for their patients.

Behavioral mechanisms behind the placebo response come down to a simple explanation: the expectation of the patient modulates the effect of drugs.

Pills

In the simplest conditioned response, pills are expected t
placebo pills bring relief because they are associated with t
medicines that have been taken before. The effects of color, size, taste,
and other attributes have also been studied in experiments that take the
subject to offer a fixed response to a stimulus, like a vending machine
that drops cans of soda when coins are inserted.

Stress

Otherwise neutral signals can serve as symbolic stresses. The cardiovascular system responds to stimuli that are important to the individual.
Bernard Lown told the story of a forty-year-old man with heart trouble.
Enrolled in an exercise tolerance testing program, the patient "observed that he was compelled each time to stop precisely after 44
crossings of the two steps." To look for a conditioned reflex, Lown
began to call out the number of times the patient had crossed the
platform. The patient consistently developed angina and electrocardiographic changes at the forty-fourth count. After a while, Lown gave a
false count, calling out "forty, forty-one, forty-two," and so forth,
when the patient reached twenty-eight crossings. At each false count of
forty-four, the man complained of chest pain, and the electrocardiographic pattern showed changes identical to those of a longer period of
exertion. When the patient became aware of the deception, he no
longer developed pain until a true count of forty-four.

"Forty-four" became a verbal clue that was responsible for the
development of the pain. Such an example of how symbols can affect
pain perception—in Lown's case, for the worse—must make us wonder at the effect of the words, comments, and attitudes of physicians
and other members of the healing professions on their patients.

Lown waited twenty years to write up this report. I conjectured that
the decision to publish might have been the result of a change in his
perception of himself—new confidence that the view of a respected
elder statesman (and Nobel Prize winner) would not be derided—or a
change in his perception of what is acceptable to editors and to the

general medical public. He responded to my query: "These experiences were so important in shaping my clinical outlook that I felt obliged to share them with colleagues. I have frequently related them in lectures. It has always been easier to present these observations to lay than to medical audiences, largely, I presume, because doctors have been miseducated and conditioned virtually to disregard biobehavioral factors. A pretentious 'scientism' mars the physicians' perception of the power of the placebo—be it word, pat, or pill." His observations fit in with some current theories about the adverse effects of hopelessness and pessimism. Beliefs can make some people sick and make other people well.

Just as anxiety worsens pain, anything that reduces or eliminates stress will relieve pain. Midbrain circuitry is the key to why. Areas in the midbrain and medulla anatomically linked to the spinal cord are important in pain perception; being chock full of opiate receptors and endogenous opioid peptides, they must have a lot to do with conditioned analgesia in animals and in humans.

Another explanation turns on richer behavioral mechanisms, the increasingly strong responses of a subject, animal or human, to repeated positive receptions of its responses. Behavior is a reaction to consequences and is therefore partially controlled by them: if you laugh when I tell a joke, I will tell another, whereas your frown may make me stop. An observer watching conditioning trials of heart rate can affect that heart rate: people caring for animals during the experimental induction of a fast heart rate evoke that quickening rate just by appearing in the laboratory. The reaction is specific to the persons involved in the studies; strangers do not evoke the same response. Heisenberg was right about the observer affecting events—or subjects.

Links between the brain and the immune system are most apparent in studies of stress, but matters grow quickly arcane. Stress is defined as "a state of disharmony that threatens the usual steady state of homeostasis." Through the nervous system and its neuroendocrine apparatus, the brain is linked to the immune system, scattered throughout the body in lymph nodes like forts, and both are controlled by the pituitary gland. Neurotransmitters—hormones pouring out from nerves—generate substances like cytokines and interleukins, which in turn affect the hypothalamic-hormonal axis. Corticotropin-releasing hormone (CRH) represents an important link between the nervous system and the immune system, for it is present in the hypothalamus of the brain and also acts directly in the periphery as an immunomodulator. CRH further attains it effects by binding to viruses or genes for inflammation or for neoplastic transformation. The purported increased survival of breast cancer patients receiving psychosocial treatment to reduce stress has been explained by this purported action.

Mechanisms are argued, but, in short, stress decreases normal cellular immune function, and that may lead to disease or to worsening of disease. The relatives taking care of a family member with Alzheimer's disease live with high levels of stress and have poorer immunological responses than people without such responsibility. A straw in the wind is worth noting: a punch biopsy wound on the forearm took nine days longer to heal in such caregivers than in others who had no such duties. Physical activity had nothing to do with the delayed wound healing; investigators thought that stress alone was responsible.

Neuroimmunology

Over the past decade neuroimmunology has opened new and exciting possibilities. The mind can translate feelings into physiological function: people die of fright or anger; burglars involuntarily defecate in living rooms they have invaded, like soldiers going "over the top"; mathematical problems derange gastric secretion; and stress can contract the gut, to pick only a few examples. To extend the control of the mind-brain to extraordinary and unusual stimuli of disease is much more difficult, even if there is a relation between stress and normal immune function and between immune function and cancer.

Like a secret service silently eliminating enemies, the immune system destroys injured tissue. The trouble is, you may corner a burglar, but you will find it hard to control a mob. There is little evidence so far that psychosocial factors influence clinically relevant measurements of immune function, as even Robert Ader, a true believer and one of the founders of neuroimmunology, lamented a few years ago.

Consider a stream at the edge of a field. It is easy to dam when the flow is gentle but far more difficult to hold back when its waters are swollen by snow or heavy rain. The raging torrents of disease are as little confined as the floods along American rivers. The nervous system and the immune system are linked, but how much they can limit the pathophysiology of disease is uncertain.

Psychoneuroimmunology has long flourished in Rochester, New York. In the 1940s researchers there associated the death of a loved one with depression of spirit and immune function. In the 1970s and 1980s Robert Ader and others showed that an immune response could be conditioned to occur with a nonimmune stimulus and, ultimately, with stress. Giving saccharin-flavored water to animals along with an immunosuppressive drug made the animals associate saccharin with the immunosuppressive agent; animals so conditioned developed a weakened immune response. After that, saccharin alone suppressed immune responses and slowed the development of an inherited auto-immune disorder: mice with the disease exposed to the conditioning stimulus lived longer than those that were not.

Conditioning lies somewhere between a simple Pavlovian stimulus response and more central authority; higher levels of the human brain do not override lower connections brought about by the repeated association of neutral events with stimulated responses. Repeated injections of a stimulant led rats to increased motor activity even after injections of plain saline, because hyperactivity had been associated with any injection. I can train my dog to fetch the newspaper by giving him a biscuit when he brings it back. Humans respond to some therapeutic situations by feeling better when they get a pill: the ritual surrounding drug administration becomes a conditioned stimulus.

Yet the physician-patient encounter should be more than a primitive conditioned response. I take the conditioning model to offer a partial, not a total, explanation of what happens when the patient receives a placebo from a physician. Only when there has been little interchange, no reassurance or plan, no engagement of the patient in self-help, does the physician-patient model parallel the criteria for a conditioned response.

Mental stimuli can affect the normal immune system, but the effects are small and require statistical manipulation for proof. Given evidence that depression inhibits the immune response, some physicians ask cancer patients to visualize their white cells and immunocytes destroying their cancer cells. These doctors often refer cancer patients to a psychologist to diagnose and treat any depression that preceded, and was possibly responsible for, the cancer.

The Role of the Physician

Conditioned regulation of the immune response is considered to parallel other pharmacophysiological effects; the doctor's office, reassurance by the physician or just the stimulus of the physician's white coat, as we have already seen, are associated with therapeutic agents and become conditioned stimuli. Repeated pairing of such stimuli with therapy lets the doctor elicit a response like that evoked by the active drug. Going to a physician makes you feel better because going to physicians before has made you feel better. A pill from a doctor, even when you are told that it is a placebo, makes you feel better willy-nilly because of your conditioned response. That may be the main reason why people with obscure pains and weakness respond so well to injections like vitamin B_{12}.

Conditioned responses act like the drugs with which they were originally linked, but morphine, paradoxically, sometimes increases pain rather than bringing the expected relief. Why that happens I do not know.

In controlled trials, any placebo effect may be strengthened by continuous reinforcement in those taking the active drug; the controls get no reinforcement because they receive only the placebo. Giving placebo and drug in varying proportions might make it possible to reduce drug dosage and side effects and even the duration and cost of therapy, or so Ader suggests. For him, "The therapeutic effect of a placebo is not something mystical, it is not a trick, and it is not a lie. As a bona fide learning phenomenon, the 'placebo effect' is amenable to experimental analysis and, rather than having been over-estimated its potential therapeutic effects have probably been under-estimated" (Ader 1995).

The central psychological state—the mind-brain—is crucial to conditioning; the doctor can make the patient receptive to suggestions on how to improve health. In animals, a previously ineffective stimulus proved effective when it was associated with food, which brought central arousal. Ader goes on: "In a sense, this may be a paradigm of the therapeutic situation where changes towards health are induced in the patient by a doctor who is able to cultivate a basic state of arousal." Patients yearn to meet their doctor's expectations because they anticipate approval and understanding.

How the conversion of medical practice from a profession to a business, and of doctors to employees of managed care corporations, will affect patients' responses to doctors and placebos remains conjectural.

To summarize, giving a placebo may evoke a conditioned reflex to the pill or to the physician. If the patient has had previous *bad* experiences with the medical system, placebos may provoke anxiety or other adverse reactions; they will not help and may even worsen the situation, acting as nocebos, not placebos. Some physicians are better healers than others, but the idea that such doctors stimulate a stronger conditioned response in patients has not received very much respect from the medical profession.

Extinction

Putting a patient in the hospital removes him or her from the setting that may have produced the illness or kept it active, and this alone may lead to improvement regardless of any other therapy. If placebos are given, they will be credited, even though removal from the stimulus has done the real work. Stopping a stimulus usually extinguishes, or at least decreases, its conditioned response, whereas repeating the stimulus reactivates those responses. People feel better on admission to a hospital because they are taken away from anxiety-provoking stimuli at home or work and because they expect to be cared for in the hospital. The relief that comes from being taken care of in a hospital is currently derided as no business of insurance companies. Patients are sent home the same day that they have given birth to a child, lost their gallbladder, or even had a breast removed. Such directives, good for profit but bad for patients, will change the positive conditioned responses into negative ones; hospital visits will be only for uncomfortable studies or therapy. It is odd that architects now try to design hospitals to make them more attractive and comforting when the patients will be discharged before they can appreciate its postmodern architecture.

Wellness Behavior

Wellness has become a popular mantra, now recited even in mainstream institutions. Based on the idea that behavioral therapy can reinforce wellness behavior rather than sickness behavior, the wellness approach aims to strengthen healthy responses instead of others that make people feel worse. In the category of sickness behavior Neal Miller lists "fatigue, weakness, various complaints, wincing, limiting physical activity, and other signs of pain." Appetite comes in eating, and placebos reinforce other wellness behavior and increase feelings of competence and control. Suggestion is an important factor. Or as Coué puts it, "Every day in every way I'm feeling better and better."

Irving Kirsch, a psychologist, is not abashed to confess that placebos work only by psychological mechanisms and are notably dependent on the patient's beliefs. He divides *expectation* into a response like joy or alertness—just the kind of emotion that one would want to enhance by placebos—and a stimulus, the money, food, or other specific reward associated with placebos. Perception is crucial to classical conditioning; a stimulus must be perceived by its effect. The response to a drug in his model is a stimulus that leads to expectancy. In that way, even a placebo response may enhance conditioning. He suggests that improvement should be noted in control trials as soon as a patient is selected for a trial, before any drug is given. Physicians will agree, for so many people relate how they feel better after just making an appointment to see a physician. So far, however, little data support any greater effect from such a promise.

Hope

"Hope helps," even if we are not yet certain that physiological changes accompany a placebo response; improvement flows from expectation. The changes are in brain activity, which might someday be pictured by PET scanning or MRI. In the depressed patient who fears recurrent depression, fear of fear can incite its reappearance, just as expectations of help from a new antidepressant enhance its effectiveness. From there, it is not far to the nocebo and the idea that pessimism hurts.

Expectation

Desire for pain relief is different from expectation of that relief, but the enumerations of desire and expectation are almost cabbalistic. Experimental subjects who are paid doubtless have happier expectations than patients suffering pain; even so, long, continued experimental pain may generate anxiety. Previous experience of past relief from analgesics affects the strength of the placebo response. Suggestion plays a role, too, along with the authority of the physician and the ceremony of the patient-physician interchange and all the other components of expectation.

The wish to be free of pain will be strengthened by the expectation that the physician will help. Postmodern doctors remember that faith, hope, and the optimistic emotions accompanying them are important. Some day it may be possible to measure emotions on a scale, to show their reality to the numerate, but for now doctors should recognize the multiple neurological, hormonal, and psychic factors that play a role in helping patients.

Compliance

Compliance—participating in a study or taking a placebo or medication that you have been advised to take—brings a benefit that not entering a study or not taking a medication lacks. Compliance is, after all, what we learned as children: good boys and girls who do what they are told will be taken care of. King and clergy gave the same message.

How well a patient follows a doctor's regimen, sometimes regardless of that regimen, has an important influence on how well the patient does. *Adherence* is a term sometimes preferred over *compliance* because it implies an equality rather than a hierarchy. Nevertheless, even for drugs that lower fat levels after a heart attack, patients who take their prescribed medication do far better than those who are less adherent, as several studies have now affirmed.

It comes down to *conditioning* and *cognition*, that last being what you think or feel. Humans may resemble rats when it comes to their neurophysiology, but how they interpret what is going on, how they view the physician or the healer, remains crucial to any consideration of placebos. That is just what must have happened in Greek temples in Aesculapian times or in miraculous shrines like Lourdes, or what may happen sometimes in a doctor's office. To give credit where it's due, however, we must return to the distinctions that philosophers, psychologists, and even physicians lose sight of in their focus on neuroimmunological mechanisms: the distinctions between illness and disease.

The meaning of the patient-physician encounter, however contorted by cultural, anthropological, and personal experiences, plays a major role in the placebo response: a satisfying explanation of the problem, expression of care and concern by the physician, and the promise of relief can enhance any therapeutic response. By taking the time, doctors can strengthen the anticipation of patients that relief will come. Listening helps, regardless of its pathways. Magic and mystery and wonder remain and can be given a push.

Mental Mechanisms

Even though very little is certain about the mental events that change brain pathways, we can recognize the placebo is a symbol of the healer's power to comfort. Injections may evoke a conditioned response, but swallowing a pill may have powerful, even sacramental, symbolic effects for a human that a rat will not feel. Pills become part of the patient, and for patients with digestive troubles, that incorporation may be very important. The sacramental power of the placebo deserves contemplation.

Gifts are symbols, too. Getting a medication from a physician is receiving a gift and a promise. For Jerome Frank, the placebo is a form of psychotherapy: "The administration of an inert medicine by a doctor to a patient is also a form of psychotherapy, since its effectiveness depends on its symbolization of the physician's healing function." For Flanders Dunbar, the right symbols have a healing aspect all by themselves, especially when they are part of a ritual, culturally accepted and readily understood; in modern times that means a pill or capsule or a ritual of some sort to stimulate self-healing mechanisms, such as an X-ray or a CT scan, both of which act as placebos even if modern doctors do not think so. In postmodern times, the placebo may even be an exercise routine, like jogging on a treadmill. Pills require little work from patients who have been educated to be passive. Alternative mechanisms seem healthier, but not everybody is ready for them, just as not everybody is ready to exercise regularly or to push away from the table.

Emphasizing the symbolic effect of placebos, psychiatrists conclude that a placebo gives patients the freedom to exercise adult functions. The placebo may function as a symbol of a loved one. "The patient becomes able to exercise his hitherto inhibited functions, but he denies his part in it, and attributes the activity to the pill. The ingestion of the pill represents a ritual or symbolic act through which one gains access to a function which otherwise remains blocked" (Krystal). Sugar pills, biofeedback machines, treadmills, a shaman's incantations, or a hypnotist's suggestions, the lure and lore of alternatives and faith—all bring benefit in much the same way: they help the patient to exercise control, to overcome an internal block.

A while ago it was reported that physicians in San Francisco did not understand why an AIDS patient felt much better even though a baboon marrow transplant had not improved his immune status. They seemed to ignore any possible placebo effect, as if all that counted were the T cells and the B cells and not the increased attention and enthusiasm and hope of the caretakers. James has his usual pertinent comment: "The medico-materialistic explanation is that simpler cerebral processes act more freely where they are left to act automatically."

Suggestion as Therapy

Modern technology is so precise that it should leave physicians more time for patients, but instead, the multiplicity of images necessitates increased communication between physicians; patients are short-circuited.

Placebos focus attention in both directions, affecting the physician who prescribes them as much as the patient who takes them. Placebos assure the patient that the physician will try to help, but they also remind the modern physician that there is a person, not just a disease, across the desk. Doctors fear therapeutic failure and may respond to their patients from their own neurotic needs: patients who do not improve threaten the doctors' professional identity and their thirst for love and admiration. Giving a placebo may lessen the intensity of that confrontation by bringing about mutual recognition of uncertainty and may even help to mobilize empathy and other helpful emotions. Giving something whose mechanisms are so baffling reminds physicians that they must be humble before their ignorance, only one person trying to help another.

Transference

Transference must play a part in the placebo effect. The emotional dependency of the patient on the physician may lead to an overvaluation of the physician and to a transfer to the physician of reactions the patient once had, as a child, to other authority figures. Analysts claim to preserve their patients' autonomy by analyzing their transference response and by not functioning as guide or model. For medical practitioners these other roles can serve a therapeutic purpose by symbolizing the continuity of the patient-physician relationship. To have patients rely on such a "magical" mechanism may diminish their autonomy, but any connection between one person and another is important in the relief of pain.

That conclusion is not so very different from James's comments about the religion of health-mindedness: "Under these circumstances the way to success, as vouched for by innumerable authentic personal narrations, is by an anti-moralistic method, by the "surrender" of which I spoke . . . passivity not activity; relaxation not intentness. . . . Give up the feeling of responsibility, let go your hold, resign the care of your destiny to higher powers. . . . a form of regeneration by relaxing, by letting go, psychologically indistinguishable from the Lutheran justification by faith and the Wesleyan acceptance of free grace, is within the reach of persons who have no conviction of sin."

In our secular age the placebo focuses the connection between patient and healer in a way that, in a more religious age, other rituals and ceremonies also did.

Attitudes and feelings about stress and helplessness are intensified by any illness. Regression to a more infantile state can be helpful or harmful; after an operation patients may help themselves by doing what they are told. Transference must have a therapeutic effect of its own, its own physiological consequences, like the claimed beneficial effects of the happier emotions. If transference is as normal a human phenomenon as its very ubiquity suggests, the merging of one human with another on a psychic level could well bring therapeutic benefit.

Transference alone may be helpful, regardless of the theory behind the therapy. There may be a direct helpfulness in the psychiatric encounter, which may be mistaken for help from the psychiatrist. Going to a doctor brings its own placebo effect; going to a psychiatrist to unburden oneself may be helpful, aside from any specific psychotherapeutic process. In large part, that is one message from controlled clinical trials.

Countertransference

Physicians' unrealistic assessment of some patients as cases of unjustified transference must also play a role in enhancing the ability of physicians to call out the internal healing power of the patient. The placebo may mobilize that healing power.

Suggestion

The discussion of transference and countertransference is a preface to my very real belief that suggestion enhances the effect of any therapy on illness; premodern doctors used to rely on it. James points out that "'suggestion' is only another name for the power of ideas, so far as they prove efficacious over belief and conduct." Mack Lipkin distinguishes *persuasion*, "influencing by argument or reason," from *suggestion*, "impressing an idea or attitude upon the mind of another by intimation." Suggestion is less obviously rational than persuasion, but they are cousins.

Paul Kaunitz, a quondam professor of psychiatry at Yale, has commented on why he offers most patients a favorable prognosis: "Positive reinforcement can foster optimism, which in turn may offer the patient a more hopeful outlook and an inducement to become well." Of the therapist he says: "It is his responsibility to influence, to the best of his ability, the patient's psychological mechanisms and external environment, so that nature's forces can bring to the fore the individual's underlying strength."

Faith, hope, and expectation are important to the power of suggestion, from going to an analyst to going to a healing shrine. Just as one physician is better at reading X-rays for reasons that may have more to do with genes than training, so others must be better at healing or comforting. One physician may give placebos with more charisma than another.

The Therapeutic Alliance

To ask the difference between a placebo and psychotherapy seems impertinent. Psychotherapists are trained, socially sanctioned healers who try to produce certain changes in their patients' emotional state, attitude, and behavior. Placebos change the perception of pain but do little to change attitudes or personality. Placebos and psychotherapeutic words alike encourage self-help and the resolution of disturbances. Placebos may function magically, whereas psychotherapy works in a more mature, rational way, but both can be part of a therapeutic alliance.

With Cousins, we can ask whether gratitude or hope or other feelings have a physiological effect and what their influence may be on the much credited endorphins. The placebo symbolizes the connection between one person and another; it locates the patient in relation to the physician, helping to form a group—something like Alcoholics Anonymous or many of the other comings together of people in a common cause. Loyalty—being seized by a commitment—is pertinent here, but I will postpone that consideration to the next chapter.

The therapeutic bond sounds very little different from a mystical religious union:

> Group-system hypothesis appears to have the advantage of parsimony and simplicity of application to fields as otherwise diverse as politics, religion, psychotherapy, and general practice. We can, for example, beneath a variety of different labels, discern the integrating force of the group system in Alcoholics Anonymous, Synanon, religious cults, faith-healing, zealous political movements, brain-washing and many forms of psychotherapy. Psychodynamic insight, psychotherapies and therapeutic communities alike provide the patient with both substitute relationships and a systematized Weltanschauung. (Adler)

The patient is swept up in a healing mode. The physiological effect of gratitude needs study: knowing that someone else is in charge, that one is being cared for, may bring healing or may encourage its start. If symbols have any physiological effect, self-help may start on its own, and self-help manuals may help those lucky enough and sensitive enough to begin to benefit from exhortations.

Even if we are not sure how placebos work, everything tells us that they help. Doctors look at the placebo as a gift from physician to patient and as a symbol of their willingness to do something. That may sound parentalistic, but the relationship between patient and physician inevitably involves one helping the other.

As Lisa Newton has put it, "I must known that the physician is in league with me against the sickness, not the other way around, or I would not consult him, and I can verify this alliance at any point during the course of treatment simply with a few minutes' conversation." She emphasizes how crucial to healing is the patient's perception of that alliance, now threatened by the role of physicians as gatekeepers or as employees of profit-making companies.

Depressive symptoms are rare in people with dependable friendships at home and at work; such people are unlikely to have persistent tiredness, anxiety, low spirits, irritability, backache, headache, palpitations, dizziness, or breathlessness. "The social environment is an important determinant of health status." Long-standing depression could be the cause of isolation, but social bonds must influence symptoms. Placebos may simply symbolize friendship and a connection, even if only with the physician as friend. Consolation has a connection with healing.

Once again, such considerations apply only to the relief of pain, suffering, or anguish. It would be outrageous for me to suggest that laying on of hands can cure diseases like cancer or heart trouble.[1] At the Health Insurance Plan of New York, in one three-year study patients who were "socially isolated and with a high degree of life stress" were four times more likely to die after a heart attack than were those with low levels of stress and lots of friends. The authors of the report suggest that a physiological mechanism—hormones stimulated by stress— evoked abnormal heart rhythms, but I do not know whether the observations have ever been duplicated. Studies suggesting such a possibility are usually wrenched out of context or selected and arranged, like the stepping stones across the river, to show a connection between two unconnected points.

Sharing one's troubled feelings, even writing them down, helps people become less vulnerable to physical illnesses, as is abundantly clear to many psychotherapists and family physicians. Confiding in someone else may protect the body against damaging internal stresses. People who are unable to share intimacies with others also have less effective immune systems. Surviving spouses of people who die suddenly and who keep their grief to themselves have more health problems than those who are able to talk about their grief. People under stress who suppress their problems have less effective immune systems than those who do not. Such observations simply give quantitative background to the old aphorism, "Sorrow that has no vent in tears makes other organs weep." We need to talk to find relief. People in psychotherapy consult physicians for medical problems less often than others do. When confiding in a spouse or a friend, one has to consider the other person's feelings and reactions, but that is not true with a therapist. A physician may help even more than a friend.

Supportive companionship can help almost anyone, although Job's comforters were chastised by God for their wavering support. One study of some interest describes how women who have already had a baby were asked to comfort other women during their first delivery. Talking, touching, and explaining what was going on reduced the percentage of caesarean deliveries from 18 to 8 percent, epidural anesthesia from 55 to 8 percent, and the like. That study suggests an emendation of the old adage "An apple a day keeps the doctor away," to "A friend a day . . . "

In disdaining placebos, modern physicians forgo the help of ritual, reassurance, and suggestion. The routine diagnostic tests that can help as placebos, if used prudently, they now turn to as suppliant rather than master. If for many, placebos are medicine's secret shame, some doctors, like Andrew Weil, unabashedly rely on behavioral changes. He labels them active placebos, including in that category meditation and relaxation techniques and, somewhat less enthusiastically, herbal medicines. All of these implicitly change mind more than body.

Takeover is the right word for the changes in medical care over the past few years, for neither physicians nor patients nor elected officials are responsible for the upheaval. Doctors have supinely accepted the new industrial metaphors of "supplier" and "consumer," along with other business terms, and have become rich, thanks in part to Medicare and the growing technological cornucopia. Still, physicians work hard, and if some have benefited to an extraordinary extent, most have labored to help their patients and have remained very much in the middle class.

The takeover came about for well-known reasons: the growing cost of medical care, the belief that a limit must be imposed on those costs, and the failure of President Clinton's health plan. That failure left a vacuum, which businesspeople rushed to fill under the pretext of controlling costs. Doctors have been converted into employees of profit-making companies, and the old-fashioned virtues praised in this book have been made obsolete; the relationships between doctors and their patients and among doctors themselves are now almost totally under the control of business interests. In this chapter I express my sorrow for what has been lost, my belief that this sorry state cannot last, and my hope that in the near future doctors and patients will again form an alliance. My tenses may mix as the past merges with the future, but that is a reflection of my passion.

What Is Loyalty?

Loyalty provides the context for placebos, a guide for the physician-patient relationship, although the term is not much favored these days.

Chapter fourteen

The

Patient-

Physician

Relation-

ship

Loyalty as

Guide

Loyalty may seem to be an antique abstraction, a professional virtue that has no meaning to modern physicians or to their remote third-party managers. Linking loyalty with placebos runs the risk of glorifying parentalism, patient dependency, and the spiritual arrogance of physicians. Yet that relationship makes giving placebos possible and, I think, ethical.

Loyalty suggests that it is not by their person alone that doctors can be faithful, but by their profession and by specific promises. Fidelity, a term sometimes heard, implies a more personal bond than the relationship between doctor and patient, which is professional by virtue of the doctor's role sworn to by those oaths of Hippocrates and Maimonides taken at graduation. Loyalty is "being faithful to one's commitments, duties, relations, associations, or values. . . . Anyone or anything to which one's heart can become attached or devoted." Loyalty need not be associated with patriotism and political allegiance alone. I associate loyalty with duty.

The Hippocratic Oath

The medical profession has had a lot to say about its duties as embodied in the Hippocratic oath. I print the oath here in full.

I swear by Apollo Physician and Asclepius and Hygieia and Panaceia and all the gods and goddesses, making them my witnesses, that I will fulfill according to my ability and judgment this oath and this covenant:

To hold him who has taught me this art as equal to my parents and to live my life in partnership with him, and if he is in need of money to give him a share of mine, and to regard his offspring as equal to my brothers in male lineage and to teach them this art—if they desire to learn it—without fee and covenant; to give a share of precepts and oral instruction and all the other learning to my sons and to the sons of him who has instructed me and to pupils who have signed the covenant and have taken an oath according to the medical law, but to no one else.

I will apply dietetic measures for the benefit of the sick according to my ability and judgment; I will keep them from harm and injustice.

I will neither give a deadly drug to anybody if asked for it, nor will I make a suggestion to this effect. Similarly I will not give to a woman an abortive remedy. In purity and holiness I will guard my life and my art.

I will not use the knife, not even on sufferers from stone, but will withdraw in favor of such men as are engaged in this work.

Whatever houses I may visit, I will come for the benefit of the sick, remaining free of all intentional injustice, of all mischief and in particular of sexual relations with both female and male persons, be they free or slaves.

What I may see or hear in the course of the treatment or even outside of the treatment in regard to the life of men, which on no account one must spread abroad, I will keep to myself, holding such things shameful to be spoken about.

If I fulfill this oath and do not violate it, may it be granted to me to enjoy life and art, being honored with fame among all men for all time to come; if I transgress it and swear falsely, may the opposite of all this be my lot.

The Hippocratic oath has come to symbolize professional loyalty to patients. Ludwig Edelstein was particular in his praise: "In all countries, in all epochs in which monotheism, in its purely religious or in its more secularized form, was the accepted creed, the Hippocratic Oath was applauded as the embodiment of truth."

Some medical students, regarding the oath as sexist and too authoritarian, have refused to repeat it even as a rite of passage. A leading critic of professional medical ethics, Robert Veatch, rather disdainfully lumps the Hippocratic oath with other professional codes of ethics, questioning "the authority of a professional group to set its own ethical standards." He finds the pledge of loyalty to the "cult group" a meaningless paternalistic promise, made by a bunch of professionals who have never discussed it with those whom they intend to benefit. Doctors have given the patient no say in those matters that really count.

But society has long acquiesced in the physician-patient relationship as one of paternalism and beneficence. Equality between patient and physician may currently be overemphasized.

The Physician-Patient Covenant

Referring to the original covenant between God and the Jews, William May likes the word *covenant* for the Hippocratic oath; it involves (1) duties to patients, (2) obligations to teachers, and (3) the setting of both in an oath to the gods.

Referrals between physicians, teaching, consultation, and daily collaboration all strengthen the bonds of loyalty between physicians. May agrees that the medical professional role is wholly gratuitous rather than responsive to the obligation that physicians owe the community for their education. Doctors cannot function without patients: "No one can watch a physician nervously approach retirement without realizing how much the physician has needed the patients to be himself or herself."

For May, a covenant provides a better model for the physician-patient relationship than a commercial contract does. A contract breaks with the authoritarian model of parent or priest in emphasizing consent rather than trust. In an equal relationship between doctor and patient, information is exchanged for goods, money for services received. A contract does not rely on charity but hardens the deal made by two people in what they take to be their own best interests.

Physicians who get up in the middle of the night to be with their patient admitted to the coronary care unit, even though the hospital staff is caring for the patient, cannot be grasping for a possible extra fee. There is more than self-interest involved, although cynics may maintain that the doctor wants to maintain control. May admits that doctors do give, but he objects to "the moral pretension of professionals who see themselves as givers alone." He wants doctors to admit that they like getting paid.

The contractual approach limits the transaction between physician and patient, specifying services for a fee and leaving no room for emergencies and contingencies. For May the ultimate solution comes in fidelity, but grounding ethics in the transcendental may not work in our modern secular and diverse society of physicians. *Covenant* carries a religious connotation that *loyalty* does not. I wonder what he would think of managed care.

Loyalty to Patients

Loyalty has not received much attention over the past several decades largely because of the evils that loyalty to authoritarian rulers has brought. Although it is no longer fashionable to talk of duty or obligation, loyalty might still provide a useful guide for medical professionals. Loyalty should suggest consideration of the doctor's role in the patient's life and death. Living wills and durable powers of attorney imply a need to protect patients against doctors. Such restraints may be necessary, but reaffirmation of loyalty might make some of them unnecessary.

Josiah Royce

Royce's *Philosophy of Loyalty*, published in 1928, has a Victorian ring to those who have lived through the era of the concentration camps, who might view untrammeled loyalty as dangerous. He defines loyalty as "the willing and practical and thoroughgoing devotion of a person to a cause. A man is loyal when, first, he has some cause to which he is loyal; when, secondly, he willingly and thoroughly devotes himself to this cause; and when, thirdly, he expresses his devotion in some sustained and practical way, by acting steadily in the service of his cause."

Loyalty is more than the captain going down with the ship. A person can be loyal by some act "which no mere routine predetermines." As an example, Royce cites the response of the Speaker of the House of Commons when Charles I came to arrest some of its members. Asked whether he saw the wanted men in the House, the Speaker answered: "Your Majesty, I am the Speaker of this House, and, being such, I have neither eyes to see, nor tongue to speak save as this House shall command; and I humbly beg your Majesty's pardon if this is the only answer that I can give to your Majesty." The Speaker had completely identified himself as the servant of a cause. Loyalty means being the willing devoted instrument of a cause or a person. "It must stir me, arouse me, please me, and in the end possess me. . . . My loyalty never is my mere fate, but is always also my choice" (Royce).

Loyalty requires an idea of community, as John Smith, one of the few modern students of Royce, explains. Scientific knowledge is not possible apart from a community with an ideal of truth. Science requires observation, evidence, validation, and a community of interpretation.

The Community of Physicians

The idea of community impels a nostalgic backward glance at the former community of physicians, with their rules, obligations, set conduct, and loyalty to the profession as a whole, as well as to each other. Maybe that community existed only in their writings or only in the eyes of their acolytes. Their community may have been a narrow one concerned with etiquette more than ethics, but at its best it provided bounds for professional and personal behavior. The training period for interns and residents instilled the notion that they were joining a community. That community may have been self-seeking—I believe it was not—but even so, it brought benefits to patients as well as physicians. Today, clinical activity is dominated by commercialism and competition, and medical practice is being pursued in the corporate spirit. As practicing doctors are banded together in groups to work for ever larger corporations, the notion of the medical profession as a calling, a community of people, appears dead or at least naive. Something must be lost, for patients as well as physicians, when that happens.

Unlike the community of doctors, the community of medical scientists, of scholars in medicine, has endured and grown. Medical scientists may be weak and not always loyal to the pursuit of truth, they may waver in hiding error or in not always searching it out aggressively, and they often defend too rigorously the failings of their own, yet they represent a true community that uplifts and sustains itself in a way that the community of practicing physicians can no longer do.

Arrogance, ambition, the craze for unlimited power, and the need for adoration are widespread among physicians, but in their work they look like a community, even if one that mingles a hope for profit with a search for truth. Many clinical organizations made up of practicing physicians may uphold the scientific ideal because science gives them their only vision of the absolute; it offers the conviction that they do make up a community. But medical practitioners today lack a sense of community, for competition is fostered in programs to cut the costs of medical care. That old clinical community might never have been quite the beloved community that nostalgia depicts, but it provided a link between physicians that provided purpose and goals and obligations to their patients.

Care of Patients

What better cause for loyalty than the care of patients? That union of passion, social utility, and intellectual interest answers Royce's question, "Is there a practical way of serving the universal human cause of loyalty to loyalty?" More than humanitarians trying to help humankind, physicians take care of the individuals before them. Their patients give them a personal, special cause. "If I am to be loyal, my cause must from moment to moment fascinate me, awaken my muscular vigor, stir me with some eagerness for work, even if this be painful work. I cannot be loyal to barren abstractions. I can only be loyal to what my life can interpret in bodily deeds."

Emotion must be involved in loyalty; the ideal physician-patient relationship has been, in contrast, more dispassionate, offering empathy, not sympathy. The emotion of physicians has been for their profession (dare I name it *calling?*) and not for their patients. Placebos can be given without commitment or emotion and still bring relief.

Loyalty in medicine could well invoke the military version, sometimes derided (outside military contexts) as obedience to higher ranks and confidence in authority figures. The notion of medicine as war, now so persuasive, used to be particularly appropriate for nursing, begun with Florence Nightingale during the Crimean War. Loyalty was the virtue for the nurse—"Loyally will I endeavor to aid the physician in his work"—and that outmoded loyalty meant refusal to criticize the hospital, training school, fellow nurses, or the physician under whom the nurse worked. I prefer to take loyalty to mean faithfulness to the patient.

Loyalty to the patient raises questions about the corporate practice of medicine, now grown so universal. It brings into focus the conflicting obligations of salaried physicians to those who hire them and to those whom they treat. It raises questions about who should enlist patients in controlled clinical trials, in which the physician in charge of the patients may put knowledge to be gained ahead of their patients' welfare. Loyalty to a patient will not permit the extra diagnostic test for a fee or the ordering of a study for defensive medicine or not doing a test that has been excluded by managed care but that the doctor thinks is essential. Thoroughgoing loyalty puts the patient's interest above all others, requires a second opinion in case of uncertainty, puts the patient above the physician or the company.

The Promise of Loyalty

A promise is "a declaration or assurance made to another person with respect to the future, stating that one will do, or refrain from, some specific act, or that one will give or bestow some specified thing." Lawyers look at a promise almost panegyrically, possibly because people breaking promises keep them busy. For lawyers, "the promise principle . . . is that principle by which persons may impose on themselves obligations where none existed before."

Contract

Lawyers like a former solicitor general have written paeans to the contract as the medium by which civilized human beings exercise their liberties. Legal contracts enforce promises, and they have three parts: promise, acceptance of that promise, and a consideration given for the promise. That consideration has to be palpable, actual, although it may be nothing more than a counterpromise, "If you do X, I will do Y."

An obligation is self-imposed, as Charles Fried sees it, and in that sense differs from a duty, defined as "an obligation owed to anyone without regard to voluntary acts and with no necessary connection with institutions or social practices." A promise is to specific persons: "We acquire obligation by promising." Promises stabilize cooperation and transactions.

In the physician-patient encounter, the physician implicitly used to say to the patient, "If you pay me, I will look out for your interests. I will do the best that I can for you." Such a promise can be more than a business contract, but it should be at least as much. Loyalty should enter into that promise. The current medical metaphors and arrangements leave loyalty out and substitute an entirely commercial relationship. Physicians work for third parties, bound only to what they have committed themselves to do, no longer loyal to loyalty. Giving a placebo should be like making a promise, with the physician telling the patient to rely not only on the physician's present sincerity but also on his or her future performance. The self-imposed obligation of service for payment received is the physician's promise of loyalty. That idea might seem to enshrine a physician-patient relationship based on private practice, but that is far from my mind. The fee sets up a continuing relationship between physician and patient. By turning over their body and their trust to a physician, patients give a second consideration, a counterpromise that they will be loyal to their physician; when patients disagree with what the physician suggests or if they intend not to work with the physician, they must say so. Patients, too, have duties and obligations that deserve more attention than they get in an era when rights are paramount. Reciprocal civility is in order.

Placebos as Promises

Placebos are as important to patients as to physicians for what they imply. The reality of the placebo response—and it is real—does not make patients passive clay in the hands of their doctors. Rather, that placebo response says that within all of us there are capacities for renewing the strength and the health of body and mind. The placebo response gives a key to self-help, whether through faith, meditation, or the Creator. The placebo effect affirms the power of community, the miracle that one person can help another simply by trying. Placebo therapy reminds us that without drugs or pharmaceutical treatment, some people can improve when their own healing powers are brought into play, whether by placebos or by practitioners of complementary approaches.

For physicians there is another message, that they, too, are human and that they can strengthen their patients by demonstrations of character, intent, and the will to help. Time builds anticipation; time with another brings healing. That states nothing new but simply recognizes the first and fundamental goal of medical care: to care and to comfort.

The physician does not promise a specific act, which would very surely lead to a lawsuit. The only promise is for some action as the patient and the physician agree on the interests of the patient.

Giving a placebo is only the first step in being loyal, but it cannot substitute for the time and energy required for devotion. A pill or another placebo may not be necessary—most of the time, will not be needed—when physicians are confident of their own therapeutic powers.

In an era when physicians were more certain of themselves, a doctor could say, "The giving of a pill by the physician to the patient is the symbol for the statement, 'I will take care of you.' " Doctors who prescribe placebos take on the obligation of loyalty. Loyal physicians can give placebos as gifts, maybe even without any more explanation than "I think this will help you," if they keep the interest of the patient uppermost in their mind. Parentalistic? Maybe, but no more so than the plumber who tells me to buy a new sink.

Giving placebos does not automatically produce loyalty or include it in the gift. There is no transubstantiation. Giving a placebo without much thought and dedication will only glorify the physician's self-image as a magic healer, able to cure without effort. That is not what placebos are all about.

The placebo has been my lens to look at science that measures and intuition that comes unbidden, at mainstream medical practice and alternative ways. Mystery can deepen understanding, and magic can spur the search for answers to forbidden questions. While science explores the universe of the cell, we may learn much about ourselves if we yield to the wonders of intuition. Someday the billions of neurons in the human brain may be traced out so that we can tape our thoughts and patch our hopes with enzymatic glues. The mind may turn out to be a program of the brain, and the Creator to be only our hope, but for now and for some time to come, our exultations rise far above their hard-wired origins.

The scientific method can be used to improve this very material world, and nowhere in these chapters should anyone find even a hint that I have turned antiscientific. Yet there remains so much that science has not conquered. Depression is cured by chemicals, but sorrow does not yield to antidepressants, nor love to antioxidants. Practitioners and patients can build the bridge between the two cultures of science and art, between perception and intuition, by looking at what alternative and holistic practitioners do and how they answer the needs of their patients.

Placebos relieve pain and heal some patients. Behavioral or mental mechanisms invoke physiological responses of endorphins, neural circuits, and immunoneurology, so the neurobiological network may bring relief. The neural cleft, that hiding place of pain-relieving agents, may provide a final common pathway by which symbols excite behavioral mechanisms—different for different

[227]

people in different places and different eras.[1] The body cannot escape the mind: our reflexes are conditioned; transference is built into us. Symbols are stimuli, each with its own message that varies over the generations. Acquired traits do not pass on through genes, but habits and reactions do pass from parent to child. Our emotional response to stimuli, whether an injection from the pediatrician or the patterns of a flag, travel through the generations. Placebos tell patients that they have a doctor who cares, and remind the doctors of the people in those bodies that they repair.

Suggestion, which plays so powerful a role in the placebo effect, should come out of the alliance between doctor and patient, but in the hurried world of modern medicine, that is not always possible. At the least, placebos stand for the doctor's promise to be loyal to the patient's best interests, but when doctors listen to patients for more than clues to disease, hearing the person who suffers and why, placebos will no longer be needed, because physicians will have learned what they once knew: that they can help to heal their patients. Placebos do not create loyalty; the physician must give it.

I do not forget the patients, who are far more than passive clay to be molded by physicians. The placebo effect and the placebo response most of all come from patients and the faith that they bring to medicine. That faith is more than priestly; it stems from the person and action of physicians and nurses, but it must be earned. In all I have said, I do not want anyone to think that the placebo effect depends only on the physician, for it is an alliance between patient and doctor alike. I have divided them for the sake of discussion.

Words as Placebos

Words can be used to exhort the healthy and the sick. Speeches may fire us to war or melt us to tears, and reassurance and comfort can mobilize healing in the sick. Words must accompany therapy if the illness of the person is to be helped. Words can be powerful placebos.

That is why so many general medical journals have opened their pages to what would have been ignored twenty years ago: poetry and narrative, philosophy and faith. That is why poetic quotations, photographs, and many other reminders of human life now find their way into the offices and clinics of doctors. Matters are changing.

Modern medical therapy has made too many physicians feel that they are mere conduits of power, of pills and procedures, helpless without technology. That misconception is reinforced by the managed care industry, which treats physicians as interchangeable modules. If physicians can regain confidence in the reality of their words, they will find once again that talking to patients and guiding them sometimes may help more than pills.

Lain Entralgo has exuberantly traced the power of the spoken word from Greek times on, but holistic and postmodern practitioners already know his message. Patients may not always be right, but they have ideas, and at the very least physicians should find out *why* their patients think they are sick. Trained to confirm observation by measurement and images, modern physicians distrust the words that reflect bodily sensations. Listening takes time, more than modern physicians claim they have, and it is far faster to look than to listen. But vision is too distant, bringing precision at the cost of intimacy. We may pray to an image, but it is not easy to talk to one.

Many people with abdominal pain of uncertain origin are studied in many ways, through every natural aperture and sometimes through artificial ones, to no avail. They may have seen a psychiatrist or psychologist and have taken tranquilizers or other pain relievers. When asked, "If you must live with this pain, will you put your head in a gas oven?" most such people reassure me that they are worried because the doctors keep doing so many tests. Few doctors nowadays ever say, "I can't explain your pain, but it won't kill you and it won't bother you forever." That reassurance from someone in authority helps.

Leo Carella wrote to me about a lesson of his early life. Tormented by a persistent ringing in his ears that no doctor could eliminate, he feared that it was going to ruin his life, until a wise old friend remarked, "I had that, too." Carella eagerly asked what he had done about it, and the man replied, "Oh, I just made the decision that it wasn't going to bother me any more. I paid no more attention to it, and told myself that I was bigger than the ringing in my ears." The simple reassurance worked. Plato's comments are still right on target:

> Sick people in the cities, slaves and free, are treated differently. The slaves are for the most part treated by slaves, who either go on rounds or remain at the dispensaries. None of these latter doctors gives or receives any account of each malady afflicting each domestic slave. Instead, he gives him orders on the basis of the opinions he has derived from experience. Claiming to know with precision, he gives his commands just like a headstrong tyrant. . . . The free doctor mostly cares for and looks after the maladies of free men. He investigates these from their beginning and according to nature, communing with the patient himself and his friends, and he both learns something himself from the invalids and, as much as he can, teaches the one who is sick. He doesn't give orders until he has in some sense persuaded; when he has on each occasion tamed the sick person with persuasion, he attempts to succeed in the leading him back to health.

Doctors today would do well to treat their patients as "free men," not slaves. Remember that doctor once meant "teacher," and doctors helped all their patients be free.

Consolation and Suggestion

Persuasion and reassurance cannot be indiscriminate, but doctors need not feel ashamed to reassure and so cheer up their patients who need some personal connection, some hope and comfort. Interest in primary care and in alternative healing practices grows from this eagerness for closer connection between patients and doctors.

Physicians and patients need to talk more about many matters: being kept from dying when cure is unlikely, getting chemotherapy for cancer, and giving away organs for transplant after death are some important issues now more widely discussed. How far to track down each complaint might also be usefully raised as a topic. Most patients go to a doctor only when they fear they are really sick; then they may want everything possible done, but some confession of humility from their doctor about what he or she can do might temper that eagerness.

How much information a patient wants merits more discussion than it elicits. If physician and patient can agree that symptom relief is enough for minor, transient complaints, much expensive and fruitless diagnostic effort might be eliminated. Unfortunately, thanks to the well-intentioned advertisements of medical institutions and physicians who promise eternal health, too many people fear that every ache or pain needs an explanation.

Not all pains come from a disease. Many are nuisances that need no inflation into plagues. I have commented on the tendency of modern doctors to elevate transient natural phenomena into diseases. When acid leaks back from the stomach into the esophagus, the heartburn that follows is easily treated with over-the-counter remedies. Studies of the sphincter that bars such reflux increased the dignity of that very common process until heartburn earned the new appellation of Gastro-esophageal Reflux Disease, or GERD, now so famed and feared. That turned a common process into an entity and gave it a reality that made marketing so-called cures easy. The imaging revolution does the same, drawing the doctor back from tolerating minor physiological blemishes into considering that everything momentarily aberrant that can be seen is a disease. I repeat what I wrote earlier, that diseases exist nowhere in Plato's sky, that they are temporary constructs of science and art, of biology and sometimes culture.

Alternative medicine looks like psychosomatic medicine to me. Psychosomatic medicine practitioners once held that diseases are affected, but not generated, by emotional, cultural, and psychological events and that physicians should treat the whole person, whose behavioral response may be as important as any more objective physiological change. Someone with rectal bleeding from ulcerative colitis, whose orifice has been poked and prodded and bathed in prescribed fluids, may worry that persistent bleeding signals a cancer lurking unrecognized. Diarrhea may rush a student from a class, but embarrassment may keep that student from returning. A politician fearing that too much responsibility is worsening his or her disease may abandon a promising career even when the physician scrutinizing only the inside of the bowel may be delighted at the patient's improvement.

Patients bring much to their disease, but modern medical training, which highlights the physician as scientist or detective, makes it difficult for mainstream physicians to feel comfortable just caring for patients or just making patients feel better. If you suggest to doctors that indigestion be relieved with the latest discovery, a proton pump inhibitor, without seeing its source with endoscopy, they will be offended that you are not scientific. Suggest that they try placebos first, and they will worry about your sanity.

By now readers may be wondering what I do believe as much as what I want them to believe. Examining placebos and the response to them has had a profound effect on me, forcing me to find room in my medical practice for mind and even spirit. Yet miracles are long gone, and although the mind, wherever it is, can control much of the normal body, disease processes gain autonomy, independent of the will and other normal controlling mechanisms. A tumor is a revolution against normal controls, disrupting the sequence of thought, will, and action so crucial to the healthy body and so very much the font of responsibility. Try as you may, after a broken neck you cannot move your arm or leg, not even a finger. The actor Christopher Reeve offers an indomitable example of how special technology can rescue an unflagging will, and he has our heartfelt admiration. Without technology or science, however, neither his bravery nor our admiration can move the smallest of his toes. Sadly, wishing does not make it so.

The Book of Job portrays the questions and answers that we all have about disease and despair, and more than a few find solace in it. The answers in Job are clear: "Canst thou draw out Leviathan with an hook? or his tongue with a cord which thou lettest down?" Only when Job has confessed his own limits does God bless his victim with more of the world's comforts than he had before. I read that lesson as a reminder that there are limits to what unaided goodwill can do.

The reader may well ask whether handing out Gideon Bibles or reprints of Job might have been easier than writing these chapters. One reason for proceeding as I have, which will not prove popular, is that I cannot ignore the publications of some professionals who go too far in their claims of what the mind can do for the ailing body. It is appropriate, laudable even, for the clergy to talk of healing, for they mean a coming together of spirit, mind, and body in a process that encourages peace of mind. That coalescence, however, does not destroy cancer or even unplug clogged arteries, however much it calms or strengthens our resolve. Humankind has achieved much against disease through technology and science and much less through thought or will or hope, or even the miracles of love.

Yet in these pages, I celebrate the miracles of hope and thought as I praise mind and spirit. Just as we tremble at some songs, weep at some stories, and are exalted by some hymns, so our courage can be strengthened and our foreboding comforted. People can learn to bear the paralysis of arm or leg, perhaps to rejoice in their burden, even though no earthly power can remove the affliction without technology and science.

I grieve that doctors who talk of healing are taking unfair advantage of their medical degrees. What was fine for Norman Vincent Peale is not appropriate for physicians who see patients in a medical setting of office or clinic and not in a temple or church. We can strengthen spirit and mind, but without medical science very little can be done for the diseased body. Contemplation of placebos has shown me the limits of what doctors and patients even together can do.

Medicine, the Silent Art

Placebos are part of medical practice, one way for the doctor to promise loyalty to the patient and a reminder that medicine is more than science. To heal, the doctor's art and person and dedication are required. As a convenient symbol for what healers can do, placebos deserve respect, but they are not as important as the patient who takes them or even the person who gives them.

Homer's physicians comforted human illness with prayer, charms, and cheering words. Later, Virgil called the medicine of his time the "silent art" because by then, physicians, fearing the irrational ways of temple priests, had abandoned songs and incantations, along with words of comfort. In the nineteenth and twentieth centuries the theories and findings of psychotherapy and psychosomatic medicine encouraged physicians to talk to their patients once again, and to listen, until the technical revolution threw medical practice back into a silence broken only by the beeps and whirs and clicks of monitors. Talk is, after all, as George Engel reminds us, "the only way patients have to acquaint their doctors with the inner experiences that made them realize that they were sick."

A colleague perplexed by a patient lamented, "I have done every possible study, and I still can't find the explanation for her abdominal pain." The patient proved to be a resident physician in a large active cardiovascular surgical service. Asked whether he had inquired into the patient's personal and emotional stresses, my friend laughed, "Howard, that's your idea. My job is to treat disease." He wanted tests, not talk, and that is what he got paid for. In ignoring the personal life of his patients, that very good and diligent physician was doing what he had been taught. Unfortunately, the case managers of managed care follow the same algorithm.[2]

Catharsis

For the most part, modern doctors pay too little attention to the release of emotions by the cathartic effect of words. Catharsis is an emotional purgation, like the effect of a tragic poem or play. "For Aristotle a physician who was able with his words to produce in a certain patient psychological effects similar to those of the tragic poem would be therapeutically more effective and complete than the one who sees therapeutic practice as only a 'mute art.' . . . Can it then be surprising that the word, an instrument so powerful and modifying in governing man's reality, should by itself, without the addition of a magical power, have the ability to achieve the cure of human disease or at least to help in it?" (Entralgo).

Hippocrates reminded doctors that "some patients, though conscious that their condition is perilous, recover their health simply through their contentment with the goodness of the physician." Surely emotions are so invigorated by poetry, music, speech, plays, and movies that the therapeutic power of words from a doctor or nurse deserves more attention. These words may change the intensity of their patients' attention and so influence their perception of their health and circumstances. Interpretation can be so helpful. Jung suggests that "a psychoneurosis must be understood as the suffering of a human being who has not discovered what life means for him. . . . The doctor who realizes this truth . . . is now confronted with the necessity of conveying to his patient the healing fiction, the meaning that quickens—for it is this that the patient longs for, over and above all that reason and science can give him."

Healing words that can bring such powerful effects need not even come from a physician. The power of presidents, preachers, performers, and poets is our daily experience. The words must be "beautiful and adequate," as Entralgo says, but for "psychotherapeutic treatment especially . . . a particular relationship must be established between the speaker and the hearer."

Doctors can and do find substitutes for words in their therapeutic programs, in rituals that they advise, and in exercise routines. Sedentary myself, I look on the endorphin rush that many joggers describe as another kind of placebo and as evidence that healing, carefully defined, can come from within. The mantras that many postmodern physicians propose offer another way of engaging the same internal strengths so helpful to so many. Different folks need different strokes, and we must find our own remedies in our own strengths.

If that is true, a physician may not be required for interpretative healing. Someone who has been through the arduous twelve years of medical training need not be the only one to encourage person-to-person healing. For hospital practice to take care of disease, prolonged training is essential for doctors to distinguish between illness and disease and to treat both. For office or clinic, however, where most patients receive their care, a wider background, in the humanities as much as in science, would be useful. Nurse-practitioners, physician-assistants, social workers, and other members of the health professions could easily care for most people in that setting. But only physicians should be trusted with placebos and then only after they have listened to the patient.

No mainstream physician will suggest that words, even heartfelt communication between physician and patient, can affect more than the attitude and emotions of the patient. Yet the relationship between the neuroendocrine apparatus of the brain and the gut helps many to imagine that attitudes in the mind, words that people hear and repeat, can affect the physiology of the body, regardless of the mechanisms. I cannot disagree with their hopes.

Empathic Listening

Empathic listening can heal, but it does not cure. The wounded healer may understand the wounded patient, but a healer who listens can help even more.[3] As someone put it, "To be human is to speak. . . . The good listener is the best physician for those who are ill in thought and feeling." Prayer comes in words to a God who listens. To heal, one must listen. The reconstruction of illness into a logical, cohesive story helps patients, but if neither doctor nor patient finds a thread, there will be only chaos.

Not all physicians and nurses are good listeners; good listeners are born more than trained. They have the capacity for caring about others who are troubled, and they can tolerate the intimacy of another's sorrow.

So scrupulously scientific a clinician as Bernard Lown writes about the lethal power of words when he tells of a middle-aged woman with low-grade congestive heart failure. She made regular visits to the clinic of Dr. Samuel Levine, a renowned Boston heart specialist. On one occasion, that noted physician announced to a group of students around the patient, "This woman has TS," and abruptly left. "No sooner was Dr. Levine out of the door than Mrs. S's demeanor abruptly changed. She appeared anxious and frightened and was now breathing rapidly. . . . I found it astonishing that the lungs, which a few minutes earlier had been quite clear, now had moist crackles at the bases. . . . I questioned Mrs. S as to the reasons for her sudden upset. Her response was that Dr. Levine had said that she had TS, which she knew meant 'terminal situation.' ''

In fact, TS stood for tricuspid stenosis, a chronic heart valve deformity. But the misunderstanding quickly led to the patient's worsening, and "later that same day she died from intractable heart failure. To this day, the recollection of this tragic happening causes me to tremble at the awesome power of the physician's word" (Lown).

As so often, Cousins phrases it well: "Words, when used by the doctor, can be gate openers or gate slammers. They can open the way to recovery, or they can make a patient dependent, tremulous, fearful, resistant. The right words can potentiate a patient, mobilize the will to live, and provide a congenial environment for heroic response. The wrong words can produce despair" (Cousins 1979).

The Therapeutic Word

My wife, Marian, tells of a visit to her dermatologist, a kind and thoughtful physician. A sportswoman much of her life, Marian played tennis and sailed in the summer and skied in the winter without much thought to the sun, which had finally taken its toll. Looking at her dolefully, her doctor moaned, "All that sun has ruined your skin." She left his office more than a little disconsolate. When she returned two weeks later, she was seen first by a young Swedish woman doctor who exclaimed, "Oh, what a wonderful outdoor face!" My wife went away enchanted, and later returned to another doctor for the latest "peeling," which comforted her in yet another way.

The therapeutic word is a reality, but outside mainstream medical practice, for the most part. Alternative practitioners know that healing has many different sources. I cannot read Hans Christian Andersen's "Little Match Girl" aloud to my grandchildren without weeping: words can surely change our perceptions.

Mainstream physicians should not be afraid to rely on suggestion in their therapy, words that can be taken in by the patient as readily as the pills so often prescribed. Words of persuasion and suggestion can address the pain, suffering, and misery of existential illnesses; doctors can reserve pills and procedures for diseases that need them more.

All of us, doctors and patients alike, receive advertisements and letters pushing new ways to lose weight, look younger, overcome heart disease, gain confidence. New books keep selling because each gives the hope that physicians no longer provide, the temporary stimulus to optimism. The authors may be entrepreneurs, but they are convincing about their healing elixirs and technological panaceas. They all promise that their new key will finally open the way to health, vitality, and longevity. Disappointment may follow, but by then a new book or therapy has appeared. From these popular approaches doctors should learn other ways to help their patients with confidence and hope.

The physician can be a vehicle for placebos.

> In this broader sense the placebo is always indicated, as a necessary adjunct to specific drugs. We often assume that compassion and experience on the part of the physician are enough, and that the fears and hopes of patients will in effect take care of themselves. Everyday life provides abundant evidence, however, that personal relationships, especially in a setting of stress, can be far more difficult—even dangerous—than many of the intellectual judgments required for proper management of patients. . . . Honest straightforward communication can relieve anxiety. Perhaps more important, this sort of placebo may make fewer and less toxic drugs necessary to produce satisfactory relief of the patient's discomfort. (Bourne)

Physicians talk of the mind-body relation, but usually treat only the body. The story that makes us weep may bring healing. If placebos can modify perceptions, tales or parables may do the same. Placebos are shortcuts, the first step in the healing process.

The Symbol of the Placebo

The placebo should be a symbol—a sacrament, I sometimes suggest —for physician as well as for patient. No substitute for clinical evaluation, it nonetheless fosters changes in the patient-physician relationship, making it focus on illness more than disease. During the ritual of history and examination, the physician can decide what is wrong and what must be done and whether—as often is true—the patient needs assurance alone. Will a diagnostic approach, dietary instructions, an exercise routine, prayer, or some other approach provide the most comfort?[4]

Thinking about placebos as sealing a therapeutic contract makes the transaction explicit. Many patients need some symbolic relief, and a placebo strengthens trust. Like the old legal seal, a prescription provides a ceremony that stops the transaction long enough to make patients and doctors think. Writing a prescription for a pill or a placebo underlines the seriousness of the contract, like pressing a ring into warm sealing wax. Doctors must trust their patients enough to prescribe placebos when appropriate, but never as a substitute for time and energy, only as the promise of loyalty.

Contemplation of the power and promise of placebos can bridge the chasm between, on one side, the rationalist basis of the medical profession and its science and, on the other, the intuitive contributions that physicians should still bring to medical practice.

We need a new term for *placebo*. It has been so disparaged and its benefits, whether psychological or physical, have been so debated that focusing on the interaction between physician and patient might be preferable to prolonging the discussion of its value. I have suggested *seal* for the legal implications of a contract, the sign of a physician's willingness to help, an icon of loyalty. Both sides to a contract have to seal the contract, so it brings real equality. In this book elsewhere I suggest *transformation*.

Placebos as Part of the Healing System

A placebo is only the first step in getting better, a small and tentative step at that, the beginning of an alliance between patient and doctor that depends on talking and listening as much as on looking and measuring. The doctor takes on an obligation of loyal care for the patient, who, in turn, should be an active and responsible partner in their alliance. Science and intuition join when placebos are given to seal the contract, prescribed by a doctor who will loyally serve.[5] There are many testimonies to the healing that comes from a strong patient-doctor relationship.

Should placebos be given for certain problems before more specific drugs? After all, some argue, if the pain of peptic ulcer or angina pectoris can be relieved by symbols that evoke healing powers or change the central perception of pain, why not use such agents, which have no real side effects, before active ones? For a particular patient I might choose a placebo; but as a matter of general policy, I must choose the more active drug. Even if peptic ulcer pain is as readily relieved by a placebo as by biologically more active drugs, healing is speeded up by acid-blocking agents, and antibiotics now cure ulcers forever.

Do doctors need to treat those 50 percent of patients whose ulcer will disappear upon scrutiny? Should they hurry along the healing? The nitroglycerine patch over the heart to relieve or prevent angina has been widely acclaimed by physicians and patients alike despite some early evidence that the effect is that of a placebo. No cardiologist would put a patch of innocent tape over the heart to relieve pain, nor would the current consensus support the idea of placebo treatment for most diseases, especially given the certainty of a lawsuit for any mishap.

Here is where alternative or complementary practitioners show so few doubts. Their different approaches, whether homeopathic remedies, exercise routines, or meditation mantras, offer rituals that strengthen the expectation of patients and so start them on the road to self-cure. I do not disparage complementary approaches by this statement, but take them as much easier and more appropriate for many.

When Should Placebos Be Used?

There is a place for placebos, a very small one: they should be used only after careful evaluation by a physician who explains and reassures and launches a diagnostic plan. Many people benefit from a tangible sign of help, even if it is just a new routine, but physicians must give more than a prescription when ordering placebos: they must promise their personal aid, for placebos are only the symbol of all that the physician does that is not quantifiable.

A placebo can be given to try to wean the addict from drugs, to relieve the patient with cancer pain before stronger agents are offered, and, with caution, to comfort the patient with pain of uncertain cause before stronger, more habituating agents are prescribed. These last are often valetudinarians, long accustomed to the behavioral benefit of a gift from the doctor. To take a broad stand against placebos for such patients seems impractical, but a placebo should never substitute for a doctor's dedication.

Yet many dedicated physicians have told how discouraged they feel when patients ask for medication after a long discussion of their problems. They are dismayed by hearing, "What are you going to give me for my pain?" Magic and suggestion may have their place in such instances, for it is as difficult for some patients to take an active role in their own treatment as it is for some doctors to let them. Who says that they should? That may sound parentalistic, but it should be obvious by now that I believe firmly in a certain degree of what used to be called paternalism, which alternative practitioners understand the value of, too.

The physician writes a prescription for the patient, predicting that the pill will help. Bloodletting, cupping, and other fancied therapeutic approaches used to serve the same symbolic function that X-rays and CAT or MRI scans and the like do today. Acute disorders have a tendency to improve, and if such pills or procedures give the physician time to decide what to do next, prescribing them is surely worthwhile. Sometimes pills take the place of a sequence of diagnostic tests to reassure patients and physicians that they are doing something. Giving an explanation and taking time to listen empathically may be just as effective, but for many, explanation is less comforting than a prescription.

Ritual plays a comforting role for most of us. The setting of the hospital or the doctor's office—what has been called the healing context—cannot be ignored. The patient who journeys to a famous clinic or physician is as ready to be helped as the pilgrim at a religious shrine. The site and circumstances of the meeting between physician and patient play important roles. Patients need an explanation for their illness consistent with their view of the world. That is best given by doctors or nurses who provide emotional support and who try to give their patients a sense of control.

Words over Pills

Some day, I hope, placebos will prove unnecessary even as a symbol of the physician's willingness to help. Placebos will serve little further purpose once physicians—and nurses, too—realize that they themselves are therapeutic, that by suggestion and persuasion, by words and little deeds, they can influence and comfort many patients. For patients, too, in that distant future, research into alternative medicine and a broadened education will help us all to realize that within us there are powers that relieve pain, counteract depression and anxiety, and heal illness. Getting a pill will no longer be necessary to trigger the responses that can come from many other sources, from meditation to massage, from prayer to pennyroyal tea. Placebos rightly given remind physicians and nurses that they are treating human beings, and assure patients that their doctor can be more than a vending machine of techniques. Once caregivers and patients see alternatives to technology and pills, both may rely more strongly on the healing alliance and the kinds of complementary practices that I have considered.

We can have it both ways, science and intuition, reason and romanticism. Both-and, not either-or. Medicine has room for both, and the dichotomies that I have set up for discussion turn out to be only parts of a whole. For the physician, there should be no split between the natural sciences and the sciences of the spirit, between mainstream and complementary alternatives. Patients are not all the same; some require more art, and some more science. Science and intuition are not mutually exclusive. The benefits of empathy and communication may sometimes be as great as the benefits of pills and potions; but when placebos help, physicians need not feel guilty at this magical side of their work, even when their patients turn to alternatives that energize mind and spirit.

I am convinced that diseases need the services of a physician. There are, alas, few proven miracles, and the slow, steady progress of scientific medicine, along with improvement in the environment and the expansion of public health services and preventive medicine, have been responsible for the improved state of health in postindustrial countries. Yet until very recently the American medical system had abandoned most other forms of healing. Illness, whether the response to pressure or the stress of having an organic disease, can be treated by healers as well as by other medical professionals. Treatment is a testimony to our common humanity, to the wonder that one person can help another and that, sometimes, we can help ourselves.

Placebos give promise of what medical practice can become in an era of technology and managed care. The physician stands between the patient and the power of modern technology; like priests of Apollo propitiating their god, modern physicians control the mysterious forces of science for the human patients whom they serve. Placebos tell us that cure depends on science and care on art but that poetry may sometimes offer the patient as much as physics, and physicians must treat despair as well as disease. The placebo differs from the computer icon, symbol of technology and power, however; it is a promise from one person to another.

In an era of imaging, placebos remind us that patients are more than their diseases, that they are people. Placebos stand for office practice, reminding us of the differences between complaints, which are very often symptoms of illnesses, and disease, which is what the hospitals are all about. To give placebos, the doctor needs only hands and a mind. Charts and images enshrine disease at a distance; they are sterile, without emotion, serene and dispassionate, and, above all, rational. Placebos are given from one to another, here and now, in a mystery that is at the same time irrational and in the romantic tradition. Icons are read by eyes. Placebos need ears. Icons may give us truth and show us disease, but placebos bring comfort. They have no power, but they bring a promise.

Interdependence, Faith, and Healing

This book is about placebos, but it is also about the universal interdependence of the human race. Most people need to belong to a group or, alas, to exclude someone else from their crowd. All of us, loners or groupies, sooner or later have to depend on others, a dependency sometimes decried as infantilism or a docility that should have been lost in growing up. Yet that ability to relax, to let oneself be cared for, to turn decisions over to others, can help the sick to heal—and does.

In so saying, I wonder whether I am turning one of my own foibles into a general rule. After all, I was a model patient, allowing my doctors to do what they thought best and suspending my judgment, something not easy for a physician. I have also been ready to accept help in other situations: if the motor on my wife's sailboat stops as we are making our way up the channel, I am the first to wave for help, whereas she, far more independent than I, prefers to do everything for herself. Who is right?

Physicians have known almost forever that part of their magic lies in caring for the patient. *Caring* is a very complex word whose meaning gets no explication here, but surely the peptic ulcer that healed when the patient came into the hospital revealed to us doctors something about the healing powers of care. What psychiatrists call group formation also helps. Men or women who bury themselves in a cause, in that loyalty praised in Chapter 14, may find their personal troubles forgotten in their new pursuit. The French Foreign Legion depended on recruits and esprit de corps for its vigor, as all armies do. Perception, the direction of attention, the expectation of feeling better—all these help people who are ill, regardless of their mechanism. That they work has much to do with the effectiveness of alternative medicine, placebos, and other practices that make the sick feel good. I have focused on placebos as surrogates for all these approaches that have a common final path. Hope helps.

On the interdependence of human beings hangs the healing of spirit and mind and the comforting of the sick body. Neurobiological pathways may run from brain to toe, but I halt at any belief that the mind can control disease. Disease is like a torrent: there is a short period when with a shovel one can dam the flow, for a stream does not turn into a torrent at once. Just so, healers and others may curb illness before it turns into disease, reverse the high blood pressure that comes from spasm, for the split between illness and disease is not so sharp.

Alternative medicine practitioners spend time with patients, talking to them and dealing with their problems in a personal as well as medical way. As psychoanalysts have come to realize, their specific rites may be less important than the time they spend and the connections they establish. Placebic communications should not be taken as sham, for different approaches have different symbolic and unexplained meanings for patients. Someone with muscle aches and pains may benefit from a massage or acupuncture, but so will someone who is lonely, and maybe even the patient with headaches. Certainly, in my own field, I would not be surprised to learn that dyspepsia can be relieved by the incantations of a shaman. After all, peptic ulcer pain is relieved by many approaches and by the right hand of fellowship.

Biomedical science, which has made many advances in medical practice, is winning its battles against the chronic diseases of cancer and heart trouble, but even so, most human complaints will not be helped by pills alone. Faith has its place.

As I pass the grand old New Haven churches now so emptied of their worshipers, I see announcement boards offering a "healing mass" or "healing service" but am uncertain whether they are affirmations of faith or help-wanted notices. The Creator, whether metaphor or Maker, no longer intervenes on our earth, or he would not have let so many innocents die in our century. But we are largely too secular and too scientifically skeptical to understand or accept a parting of the seas or walking on the water. Manna may have fallen from the skies, and the loaves and fishes multiplied, but in our time public health officials would forbid their consumption without extensive prior testing. That is why I am more than a little surprised to find postmodern physicians gossiping about what prayer and hope can do for cancer. I assume they mean what it can do for their patients with cancer.

The modern loss of faith leaves us yearning for visions of paradise lost, and people search in the desert for the floodgates of love and comfort. The lowly miracles of our time, placebos and alternative medicine, faith-healing—you name it—stand for the comfort that healers can bring, but they do not cure even when they heal. Still, healing can be ours with individual and concerted will and goodwill. Healing comes from the Creator, mind and spirit. But cure comes only from science and technology.

Notes

chapter one
Introduction

1. *Complementary medicine* is a more appropriate term than *alternative medicine* because it includes such supplemental measures as relaxation therapy and nutritional advice. Respected physicians like Herbert Benson and Andrew Weil, both graduates of Harvard Medical School, would not claim that their methods supersede mainstream medicine but rather that they supplement and only occasionally replace it.

chapter two
The Placebo Drama

1. A pervasive issue is whether placebos have an effect on disease or whether they just make patients feel better by relieving symptoms. Because the borders between disease and illness are so fuzzy, there is as yet no sharp answer. Some observers distinguish between the *specific* effects of placebos, which might account for some miraculous cures, and those more *nonspecific*. They argue that a placebo that looks like an active agent might bring about the same benefits as does the active agent that it mimics, a thesis that needs proof. If a person has been taking antacid medications for years, substitution of an inactive identical gel would presumably relieve dyspepsia as a specific effect, the nonspecific effects remaining subsumed under hope and adherence to the therapeutic program. My theme throughout this book is that hope helps; my difference with other proponents of placebos and alternative medicine lies in the strength of that help.

2. A. K. Shapiro deserves the proverbial lion's share of credit for reviving the concept of placebos, but Henry Beecher, one of my teachers at Harvard Medical School, also contributed enormously. Because Shapiro was a psychoanalyst and Beecher an anesthesiologist, both dealt with the unconscious.

3. Charles Moertel of the Mayo Clinic and I years ago set up the GI Tumor Study Group to improve therapy for patients with

gastrointestinal cancers. Following statistical niceties, we required a certain minimum number of patients at each cooperating institution. As it became clear that physicians were dragooning patients into the studies in order to clear that hurdle of the "body count," I began to worry about how often physicians talked patients with cancer into joining a trial out of less than generous motives. That concern deserves more discussion than it gets.

4. "Don't just stand there; do something" is an old rule for physicians; the cynical add, "Before the patient gets better." Most minor problems go away on their own, but even postmodern physicians find it hard to understand that not all aches and pains need treatment or diagnosis. Now that special interests are publicizing "disease management"—known to the trade as "carve-outs"—to urge a sequence of diagnostic tests that just happens to serve their profit-making ventures, therapeutic triumphalism will win out over watchful waiting.

5. Some have suggested that I may go too far in my praise of intuition. Yet many stories make me sure that one person can help another by wanting to and by taking the time to try. This is not just an old man's idea; in the first (1970) edition of my textbook *Clinical Gastroenterology*, I wrote about the "will to cure" (p. 608)—how sitting down with a patient to focus on that person's situation provided an essential part of the treatment for colitis.

chapter three
The Physician

1. Any distinction between intent and belief seems less important to me now than earlier, for I have come to consider what the doctor or pill does less important than how the patient reacts. Even so, enthusiasm that stems from the faith of the physician also has a legitimate role. Does that mean that religious physicians should pray with patients? A Congregational minister once complained to me that his born-again physician hummed "Amazing Grace" as he was sigmoidoscoping him. Some believing physicians do not find it amiss to share a prayer of hope or thanksgiving with those of similar religious beliefs, even in the office.

2. I write this in 1998, when managed care drains vast sums of money that should have gone to the care of the sick into the pockets of shareholders. The changes are so kaleidoscopic that no one can predict how legislative regulation and the anger of an aroused public will shape the medical care system of the future.

3. In an ideal world, everyone would have a family physician, whether

nurse-practitioner, physician-extender, or more lengthily trained physician. My nurse-practitioner daughter, Martha, claims that doctors remain captivated by disease and technology, whereas nurses prefer listening to their patients. Still, for patients sick enough to be in a hospital, specialists offer better, if more intensive and expensive, care than family physicians, who should be in an office or clinic or visiting a patient at home. Years ago, Harvey Mandell and I suggested that young physicians fresh out of training should be the hospital specialists; older doctors, over sixty, are better family doctors because they have had more experience, which makes for understanding, empathy, and patience.

4. When I was writing this, a retired professor of classics complained that his surgeon had removed what needed to go but had not warned him to expect severe postoperative pain for a few days. Worry about persistent pain drove him to a hospital emergency department—a trip that might have been prevented by a few words.

5. Disease management practices, known to doctors as algorithms, focus on specific diseases and how they should be treated; algorithms ignore the many varieties of patients who can have the same disease. To lay out specific steps for treatment is to highlight the disease and ignore the preferences or general condition of patients. My professional gastroenterological organizations have been pressing to ensure that colonoscopies be adequately paid for, a crusade that confuses instruments with doctors. Doctors themselves have not yet asked to be paid to spend more time with their patients except at one orifice or another.

6. Nikola Biller, whom I thank in my Preface, pointed out to me the mother-child metaphor that feminists are now bringing into medicine. That model, which deserves more explication by men as well as women physicians, can be read about in Virginia Held's papers.

chapter four
Pills and Procedures

1. Not all dyspepsia requires medical attention. My grandfather, like most others of his time, happily took baking soda—"saleratus"—for occasional indigestion. Today he would run the risk of having a scope thrust down his throat to check for all kinds of dire diseases of the gullet that he might never have had.

2. An active clinician at mid-century, Mack Lipkin, who had many psychiatrists as patients, thought a lot about the benefits of placebos. I plundered his collection of ideas on a visit to his home in North Carolina a long time ago, and I am still grateful to him. His son, Martin, also a doctor, maintains an interest in patient-physician relationships.

3. Women suffer many more gastrointestinal complaints than men, doubtless for purely physiological reasons, a situation that many ascribe to their subordinate position in a patriarchal society. What happens to the next generation may answer that question.

4. To equate many alternative medicine approaches with placebos does not disparage them. Postmodern physicians, more eclectic than an earlier generation of doctors, recognize how much hope helps. Many premodern clinicians knew that the color of a pill may enhance its pharmacological or placebic effects, as may its very name. In the 1950s Eskay's Neurophosphates was the name of a tonic, made more efficacious when pronounced emphatically.

Ann Harrington of Harvard finds seven themes at the core of the mind-body relation. Connection counts the most, I think; when a person no long feels alone or isolated. That is what placebos, or a positive attitude, are all about. Human beings are not solitary, as Adam's lament to his Creator tells us.

chapter five
The Patient and the Disease

1. Others will argue that comforting an ill patient, no matter how, helps the disease that often enfolds illness. We need a term for those borderlands, the unclaimed land between disease and illness. Irritable bowel lies in that never-never land, but because it has at least a hundred years of history behind it, most doctors accept it as a definitive syndrome with physiological but no anatomic traces. Many physicians have more trouble with chronic fatigue syndrome and posttraumatic stress syndrome.

2. Anatole Broyard, the well-known literary critic, was saddened by modern medical practices because of his encounters with a number of Boston area physicians who treated his prostate cancer but paid less attention to him.

3. The two approaches to depression need not be incompatible. The serotonic re-uptake system could be deranged by genetic arrangements and thus especially susceptible to emotional or psychic stress.

4. Hayden Pelliccia gave me this phrase, which neither he nor I have been able to trace. If anyone knows its provenance, do let me know.

chapter six
What Placebos Can Do

1. The experiments were done with varying consistency in terms of whether the patients were told about possible side effects or benefits. So far as I know, no one has attemped to prevent the side effects of a placebo with another placebo, except in Irving Kirsch's studies at the University of

Connecticut. Herbert Benson's "relaxation response" might be an ideal technique for such a study.

2. This report has been accepted unchallenged to a mind-boggling extent as an example of what placebos can do. I find a certain poignancy in this tale because Andrew Ivy was the sponsor of krebiozen, now long considered a worthless agent. He was a noted gastrointestinal physiologist, whom I much admired, and a medical consultant at the Nuremburg trials of Nazi doctors.

3. Rose Papac, a sophisticated Yale oncologist, gives an up-to-date account of spontaneous regression of cancers.

4. I ignore here a number of other controlling mechanisms and inflammatory agents, like the cytokines, which are immunomodulators as well as neurotransmitters. To consider them in detail would lead us too far astray and would not significantly affect my main argument.

5. A patient with fibromyalgia, for example, may improve on a regimen that enlists his or her fighting spirit. Patients who participate in an advocacy group often lose their complaints. In the 1960s, some of my patients abstained from drinking for long periods when they joined the Black Panthers. I ascribe their abstinence to that new allegiance and turn to Josiah Royce's words on loyalty (Chapter 14).

chapter seven
Patients and Pain

1. The neurological network is something like a series of electric train tracks, which must be joined together for neurotransmitters such as serotonin to pass along the nerves and activate pain fibers. When the neurotransmitters are confined to their site of origin, pain is relieved. Doctors try to be very precise about pain as a signal of something worse. The adjectives that the patient chooses are less important than when the pain comes and goes or what makes it better or worse.

2. A legendary patient thought he was dying when his longtime heartburn was relieved by the new H2-blockers: he worried that the fire in his belly fed the steam engine that had kept him going, and if it died, so would he.

3. Any physiology textbook will give far more details than are found here. The point is that pain is more than a sensation in the brain following a pinch of the skin. It is more like polyphonic music, a symphony meant to be heard, its chords and cadences bringing almost physiological responses. Just as certain chords require yet another chord to satisfy the hearer, so pain is interpreted differently by different people in different circumstances.

4. Endorphins are no more reliably measured now than earlier. Most current

studies look at perception, for techniques for measuring endorphins are too imprecise.

5. Where I differ from Benson, Weil, and other acclaimed practitioners is in my skepticism about how far the effect of hope or faith can go in lessening functional problems that have caused anatomic derangement of permanent structural alterations. Others proclaim that hope is far more powerful than to be stumped by anatomical infelicities. At Lourdes, however, only one in forty thousand miracles is said to be certified by the Catholic Church, so I wonder how much more the secular physician-healers can promise their adherents.

chapter eight
Autonomy and Responsibility

1. Ivan Illich, variously a Marxist, a Jesuit, and a world traveler but always a social critic, has many incisive opinions about modern society, all recounted in his book *Medical Nemesis*, published first in Great Britain in 1975 and recently republished.

2. Doctors are the worst of all ageists; in their daily work they meet the weak and the sick. The old are more likely than the young to be frail, confused, and in need of help, so it is understandable that doctors conflate sick and confused elderly patients with all old people.

3. These stories are examples of pathography, which, like narrative in general, now has great influence on medical thinking. Pathography is the story of the illness in the patient, sometimes told by the patient and sometimes by a physician to teach other doctors. Ann Hawkins has likened them to the conversion accounts of seventeenth-century America. Many stories of illness end up as parables with varied interpretations. Even medical ethicists are returning to storytelling, which they call casuistry. As accounts of medical truth, however, anecdotes are still derided, even though something that has happened once is likely to happen again.

chapter nine
Objections to Placebos

1. Ethicists display options, showing how they can be justified and what their consequences would be. Physicists look for natural laws but do not invent them—quite a different activity from what ethicists can do in the absence of a consensus about revealed Truth.

2. Old people learn that the body they once took for granted demands ever more attention, and so do sick people. Once when I was lamenting the frailties of age and the unreliability of the body, a young woman responded, "But that is what it is like to have ulcerative colitis."

3. Here I borrow the persuasive arguments of Allan Buchanan.
4. Finding a disease in a ''presymptomatic'' person puts that newly minted patient under a cloud. A woman of seventy-five warned of a high cholesterol count and given a rigid diet and pills to improve her statistical chances of living longer may be less comfortable than one who knows that her mother lived to one hundred and who has never heard of cholesterol, hard though that may be to imagine. People over seventy used to die without guilt, but no longer; no one outlives the call for prevention by early detection. Only a few diseases can be prevented; for instance, the avidity of the liver for iron, hemochromatosis, one of the commonest genetic faults in white males, can be prevented by taking away a pint of blood on a regular basis. Looking for a symptomatic coronary artery disease does not yet fall into the same category.
5. James Fixx, the well-known physician-writer who made running a national pastime, exercised strenuously yet died early of cardiovascular disease, which made his followers rejoice that he would have died even younger had he not run so far and so often.
6. Here I rely on Kapp's magisterial account.

chapter ten
Alternative Medicine
1. Here I rely on Lynn Payer's account of how medical practices and customs differ from one country to the next.
2. The idea that the mind can improve the ailing body leads to guilt if there is no improvement, particularly if the patient has been convinced that depression precedes cancer by lowering immune activity. The narcissism involved in eating for health alone may curtail the festivity of banquets and other happy occasions.
3. Dan Ullman, president of the Foundation for Homeopathic Education and Research, is quoted as saying, ''Homeopathy is a different system of treating people. . . . It doesn't treat diseases per se, but treats people who are ill'' (*JAMA*, October 19, 1994, p. 1156). As a British physician, Thurston Brewin, has put it, sick people hope for ''more attention, more time, more sympathetic understanding, more hope,'' and they get that from attentive physicians.

chapter eleven
Placebos, Alternative Medicine, and Healing
1. That miracles always happen elsewhere makes them hard to evaluate or accept without resources or much experience of them.
2. Studies are planned on the efficacy of prayer in healing by Herbert Benson

in Boston. He may not have been convinced by the claims of transcendental meditators that prayer can influence the stock market and even the growing of crops.

3. Unless Samuel Hahnemann and his followers have discovered some new law of physics, homeopathic remedies are clearly empirical only—handed down but never tested. At best, their routines call for painstaking discussion with patients, including emotional and psychological factors. That faith in the ear contrasts sharply with the mainstream practitioner's reliance on the eye and the images so readily but so expensively obtained.

4. Carol Bayley describes in some detail arguments between distinguished scientists about the effectiveness of homeopathic drugs.

5. In defending a wider approach than the usual Eurocentric view common at Yale, a dean pointed out that a poem by Keats, for example, has taken on so much more meaning for students than one by a poet from the third world because of the energy put into its scrutiny over the past 150 years. That observation is not far from Harold Bloom's thesis that readers bring as much to a poem as its author. Those who follow a hundred years later feel the influence of poets yet unborn when the poem was written. In the same way, the faults of alternative medicine are highlighted by proponents of orthodox approaches, but the same scrutiny is not always afforded the reported mainstream medical successes.

chapter twelve
Why Doctors Don't Like Placebos

1. In this chapter I borrow heavily from the work of Isaiah Berlin and Arturo Castiglione, and doubtless many others, who have been so persuasive that I have taken their ideas for my own.

2. Talk of charlatans and their hidden ways may make some think about the reputed secrecy at the Sigmund Freud Archives. Psychoanalysis, banished now to literary and philosophical circles, may have adopted some trappings of a cult. Asking if iridology practitioners deserve a slice of medical care costs is not equivalent to turning a deaf ear to the paeans to psychoanalysis.

chapter thirteen
How Placebos May Work

1. If psychosocial factors are so important in the pathogenesis of pain and suffering and illness and all the emotional correlates of disease, it may not be outrageous to suppose that they might play an equal role in the pathogenesis of disease itself. The laying on of hands once helped people with many troubles and still could, but such an approach has never

helped cancer. These issues can be clarified with a better delineation of disease and illness. Until then, maybe that old word *disorder* might provide neutral ground.

chapter fifteen
The Promise of the Placebo

1. In emphasizing the important role of culture in the construction of disease, Robert Aronowitz contrasts Lyme disease, described in the United States as a disease defined by arthritis, with the same disease in Europe, where as *erythema chronicum migrans* it becomes a concern of the dermatologist.
2. Doctors are especially reluctant to talk about personal problems with a sick colleague. Sick physicians are given the courtesy that speeds up the needed tests but with a reserve that avoids any emotional issues that might embarrass the doctor-patient or doctor-doctor in the future.
3. I like the phrase, "the listening healer" and borrow it from Stanley Jackson, a friend who has used it in his marvelous essay *The Listening Healer*.
4. Some physicians may take this to mean that nobody ever needs a diagnostic workup. That is not so; but illness is part of disease, and most patients want empathy and comfort as well as science.
5. What will the new employee status of most physicians in a managed care system portend for a doctor's loyalty? Because I cannot believe that for-profit managed care will long endure, I pass over the problem as temporary. Salaried employees—whether physicians or nurses—of a not-for-profit institution, like the military or university hospitals that I have worked in, can offer loyal care.

I have so far been a patient on two occasions, lucky to have others advise and make decisions for me because I have been cared for by those who know me, a doctor sick in his own hospital.

Works Cited

Ader, R. The psychoimmunology of cancer. (Book review.) *JAMA* 344:1489–1490, 1994.

Ader, R., and Cohen, N. Psychoneuroimmunology: interactions between the nervous system and the immune system. *Lancet* 345:99–100, 1995.

Adler, H. M., and Hammet, V. O. The doctor-patient relationship revisited: analysis of the placebo effect. *Ann. Intern. Med.* 78:595–598, 1973.

Alderman, M. H. Non-pharmacological treatment of hypertension. *Lancet* 334:307–311, 1994.

Alexander, F. Functional disturbances of psychogenic nature. *JAMA* 100:409–473, 1933.

———. *Psychosomatic medicine*. New York: Norton, 1950.

Alternative medicine: expanding medical horizons. National Institutes of Health publication 94:066. December 1994.

Apkarian, A. V. Functional imaging of pain: new insights regard the role of the cerebral cortex in human pain perception. *NeuroSciences* 7:279–293, 1995.

Aronowitz, R. Lyme disease: the social construction of a new disease and its social consequences. *Milbank Quarterly* 69:70–112, 1991.

———. *Making sense of illness: science, society, and disease*. New York: Cambridge University Press, 1998.

Aronowitz, R., and Spiro, H. The rise and fall of the psychosomatic hypothesis in ulcerative colitis. *J. Clin. Gastroenterol.* 10:298–305, 1988.

Asai, A., Fukuha, Ra S., and Lo, B. Attitudes of Japanese and Japanese-American physicians towards life-sustaining treatments. *Lancet* 346:356–359, 1995.

Barrett, R. J., and Lucas, R. H. Hot and cold in transformation: is Iban medicine humoral? *Soc. Sci. Med.* 38:383–393, 1994.

Barrett, S. The public needs protection from so-called alternatives. *Internist* 35:10–11, 1993.

Barsky, A. J., and Borus, J. F. Somatization and medicalization in the era of managed care. *JAMA* 274:1921–1934, 1995.

Baumer, F. L. Romanticism. In *Dictionary of the history of ideas*, vol. 2, ed. R. P. Wiener. New York: Scribner, 1973, pp. 198–204.

Bayley, C. Homeopathy. *J. Med. Phil.* 18:129–145, 1993.

Beecher, H. K. The powerful placebo. *JAMA* 159:1602–1606, 1955.

———. Surgery as placebo. *JAMA* 176:1102–1107, 1961.

Benson, H. *Timeless healing*. New York: Simon and Schuster, 1996.

Benson, H., and McCallie, D. P. Angina pectoris and the placebo effect. *New Eng. J. Med.* 300:1424–1429, 1979.

Berger, J. T. Placebo use in patient care: a survey of medical interns. Unpublished MS.

Bergson, H. *Creative evolution*. New York: Modern Library, 1944, p. 194.

Berkowitz, C. D. Homeopathy: keeping an open mind. *Lancet* 344: 701–702, 1994.

Berlin, I. *Against the current*. New York: Penguin, 1980.

———. The counter-enlightenment. In *Dictionary of the history of ideas*, vol. 2, ed. R. P. Wiener. New York: Scribner, 1973, pp. 100–112.

Binder, H. J., Cocco, A., Crossley, R. J., et al. Cimetidine in the treatment of duodenal ulcer. *Gastroenterology* 74:380–388, 1978.

Black, P. H. Psychoneuroimmunology: brain and immunity. *Science and Medicine* 2:16–25, 1995.

Blackwell, B., Bloomfield, S. S., and Buncher, C. R. Demonstration to medical students of placebo responses and non-drug factors. *Lancet* 1:1279–1282, 1972.

Blum, A. L. Is placebo the ideal anti-ulcer drug? In *Peptic ulcer disease*, ed. G. Bianchi and K. D. Bardhan. New York: Raven Press, 1982, pp. 57–61.

Blum, R., and Blum, B. *Health and healing in rural Greece*. Stanford: Stanford University Press, 1965.

Bok, S. The ethics of giving placebos. *Scientific American* 231:17–22, 1974.

———. *Lying: moral choice in public and private life*. New York: Pantheon Books, 1978.

Bond, M. *Pain: its nature, analysis and treatment*. New York: Churchill Livingstone, 1979, p. 135.

Bonhoeffer, D. Ethics, ed. E. Bethge. New York: Macmillan, 1962, p. 326.

Bonser, W. *The medical background of Anglo-Saxon England*. London: Wellcome Historical Library, 1963, p. 211.

Bourne, H. R. The placebo: a poorly understood and neglected therapeutic agent. *Rational Drug Therapy* 5:1–6, 1971.

Brand, P., and Yancey, P. *Pain: the gift nobody wants*. New York: Harper Collins, 1993.

Brewin, T. B. Three ways of giving bad news. *Lancet* 337:1207–1209, 1991.

Brewin, T. Logic and magic in mainstream and fringe medicine. J. Roy. Soc. Med. 86:721–723, 1993.

Brodhead, R. H. An anatomy of multiculturalism. Yale Alumni Magazine 57:45–49, 1994.

Brody, H. The lie that heals: the ethics of giving placebos. Ann. Intem. Med. 97:112–118, 1982.

———. Placebos and the philosophy of medicine. Chicago: University of Chicago Press, 1980.

Brown, W. A. Placebo as a treatment for depression. Neuropsychopharmacology 10:265–269, 1994.

Broyard, A. Intoxicated by my illness. New York: C. Potter, 1992.

Buber, M. The William Alanson White Memorial Lectures, fourth series: distance and relation. Psychiatry 20:97–113, 1957.

Buchan, D. The writings of David Rorie. Edinburgh: Canongate Academic, 1994.

Buchanan, A. Medical paternalism. J. Philos. Pub. Affairs 7:370–390, 1978.

Buchman, R., and Lewith, G. What does homeopathy do—and how? Brit. Med. J. 309:103–106, 1994.

Budd, M. A. and Gruman, J. C. Behavioral medicine: taking its place in the mainstream of primary care. HMO Practice 9:51–52, 1995.

Burt, R. A. Taking care of strangers. New York: Free Press, 1979.

Busbaum, A. Memories of pain. Science and Medicine 3:22–31, 1996.

Byck, R. Psychological factors in drug administration. In Clinical Pharmacology, ed. K. Melman and H. Morelli. New York: Macmillan, 1978, pp. 110–126.

Byerly, H. Explaining and exploiting placebo effects. Perspectives Biol. Med. 19:423–436, 1976.

Bynum, W. F. Medicine and the five senses. New York: Cambridge University Press, 1994.

Cabot, R. C. Suggestions for re-organization of hospital out-patient departments. Maryland Med. J. 50:81, 1907.

———. The use of truth and falsehood in medicine, ed. J. Katz. Conn. Med. 42:189–194, 1978.

Cabot, R. C., and Dicks, R. L. The art of ministering to the sick. New York: Macmillan, 1947.

Cahoone, L., ed. Modernism to postmodernism. Cambridge: Blackwell, 1996.

Camp, V. The place of acupuncture in medicine today. Brit. J. Rheumatology 39:404–406, 1995.

Cannon, R. O. The sensitive heart: a syndrome of abnormal cardiac pain perception. Jama 273:883–887, 1995.

Cannon, W. B. Gains from serendipity. In *The way of the investigator*. New York: Norton, 1945.

Carella, L. Personal letter, 1995.

Carey, T. S., Garrett, J., Jackson, A., et al. The outcome and costs of care for acute low back pain among patients seen by primary care practitioners, chiropractic practitioners, or orthopaedic surgeons. *New Eng. J. Med.* 333:913–917, 1995.

CASS principal investigators. Coronary artery surgery study (CASS), a randomized trial of coronary artery bypass surgery. *Circulation* 68:939–950, 1983.

Cassell, E. J. *The healer's art*. New York: Penguin, 1976.

————. The nature of suffering and the goals of medicine. *New Eng. J. Med.* 306:637–645, 1982.

Cassileth, B. R. Survival and quality of life among patients receiving unproven as compared with conventional cancer therapy. *New Eng. J. Med.* 324:1180–1185, 1991.

Cassileth, B. R., Lusk, E. J., Miller, D. S., et al. Psychosocial correlates of survival in advanced malignant disease? *New Eng. J. Med.* 312:1551–1555, 1985.

Castiglione, A. *A history of medicine*. New York: Knopf, 1947, pp. 148–178.

Chakraborty, A. Culture, colonialism, and psychiatry. *Lancet* 337:1204–1207, 1991.

Chrousos, G. P., and Gold, P. W. The concepts of stress and stress-systems disorder. *JAMA* 267:1244–1252, 1992.

Clouse, R. E. Anti-depressives for functional gastrointestinal syndromes. *Dig. Dis. Sci.* 39:2352–2363, 1994.

Clouser, K. D., and Hufford, D. J. Non-orthodox healing systems and their knowledge claims. *J. Med. Phil.* 81:101–106, 1993.

Cobb, L. A., Thomas, G. I., Dillard, D. H., et al. An evaluation of internal-mammary-artery ligation by a double-blind technique. *New Eng. J. Med.* 260:1115–1118, 1959.

Cohen, S., Doyle, W. J., Skoner, D. D., et al. Social ties and susceptibility to the common cold. *JAMA* 277:1940–1944, 1997.

Commentaries. *Neuropsychopharmacology* 10:271–288, 1994.

Connelly, D. M. *Traditional acupuncture*. Columbia, Mo.: Center for Acupuncture, 1975.

Cousins, N. Anatomy of an illness (as perceived by the patient). *New Eng. J. Med.* 295:1460–1463, 1976.

————. *Anatomy of an illness as perceived by the patient*. New York: Bantam, 1979.

————. *The healing heart*. New York: Norton, 1983, p. 135.

Cross, S. E. Pathophysiology of pain management. *Mayo Clin. Proc.* 69:375–383, 1994.

Davidoff, L. What one neurosurgeon does. In *Should the patient know the truth?* New York: Springer, 1955, pp. 88–92.

Davies, G. The hands of the healer: has faith a place? *J. Med. Ethics* 6:185–189, 1980.

Dawson, J. P., Harvey, W. B., and Henderson, S. D. *Contracts.* Mineola, N.Y.: Foundation Press, 1982.

DeCrean, A. I., Roos, P. J., DeVries, A. L., et al. Effect of colour of drugs. *Brit. Med. J.* 313:1624–1626, 1996.

DeDombal, F. T., Leaper, D. J., Horrocks, J. C., et al. Human and computer-aided diagnosis of abdominal pain: further report with emphasis on performance of clinicians. *Brit. Med. J.* 1:376–380, 1984.

Desharnais, R., Jobin, J., Cote, C., et al. Aerobic exercise and the placebo effect. *Psychosom. Med.* 55:149–154, 1993.

DeVita, V., Hellman, S., and Rosenberg, S. A. *Principles and practices of oncology.* 5th ed. Philadelphia: Lippincott-Raven, 1997, pp. 2993–3001.

Dimond, E. G., Kittle, C. F., and Crockett, J. E. Comparison of internal mammary ligation and sham operation for angina pectoris. *Amer. J. Cardiol.* 5:483–486, 1960.

Dobrilla, G., and Scarpignato, C. Placebo and placebo effect: their impact on the evaluation of drug response in patients. *Dig. Dis.* 12:368–377, 1994.

Dollery, C. T. A bleak outlook for placebos (and for science). *Eur. J. Clin. Pharmacol.* 15:219–221, 1979.

Dunbar, F. Emotions and bodily changes. 4th ed. New York: Columbia University Press, 1954.

———. *Psychiatry in the medical specialties.* New York: McGraw-Hill, 1959.

Edelstein, L. Appendix (letters from William James to William Osler). *Bull. Hist. Med.* 20:292–293, 1946.

———. *The Hippocratic oath: text, translation and interpretation.* Baltimore, Md.: Johns Hopkins University Press, 1943, p. 64.

———. The professional ethics of the Greek physician. *Bull. Hist. Med.* 30:391–419, 1956.

Egbert, L. D., Battit, G. E., Welch, C. E., et al. Reduction in post-operative pain by encouragement and instruction of patients. *New Eng. J. Med.* 270:825–827, 1964.

Eikelbaum, R., and Stewart, J. Conditioning of drug-induced physiological responses. *Psychological Rev.* 89:507–528, 1982.

Eisenberg, D. Advising patients who seek alternative medical therapies. *Ann. Intern. Med.* 127:61–69, 1997.

Eisenberg, D. M., Delbanco, T. L., Berkey, C. S., et al. Cognitive behavioral techniques for hypertension: are they effective? *Ann. Intern. Med.* 118:964–972, 1993.

Eisenberg, D. M., Kessler, R. C., Foster, C., et al. Unconventional medicine in the United States: prevalence, costs, and patterns of use. *New Eng. J. Med.* 328:246–252, 1993.

Eisenberg, L. Disease and illness: distinctions between professional and popular ideas of sickness. *Culture, Medicine, and Psychiatry* 1:9–23, 1977.

———. A friend, not an apple, a day will keep the doctor away. *Amer. J. Med.* 66:551–553, 1979.

———. Treating depression and anxiety in primary care. *New Eng. J. Med.* 326:1080–1084, 1992.

Engel, G. L. How much longer must medical science be bound by a seventeenth century world view? *Psychother. Psychosom.* 57:3–16, 1992.

Entralgo, P. L., Rather, L. J., and Sharp, J. M., eds. and trans. *The therapy of the word in classical antiquity.* New Haven: Yale University Press, 1970.

Epstein, A. L., Budd, M. A., Cole, S. A. Behavioral disorders: an unrecognized epidemic with implications for providers. *HMO Practice* 9:53–56, 1995.

Ernst, E. The power of the placebo. *Brit. Med. J.* 313:1569–1570, 1996.

Everson, T. C., and Cole, W. H. *Spontaneous regression of cancer.* Philadelphia: Saunders, 1966, p. 4.

Fabrega, H. The need for an ethnomedical science. *Science* 189:969–975, 1975.

Feinstein, A. R. Should placebo-controlled trials be abolished? *Eur. J. Clin. Pharmacol.* 17:1–4, 1980.

Feyerbend, P. *Against method: outline of an anarchistic theory of knowledge.* London: Verso, 1978.

Fields, H. L. Neurophysiology of pain and pain modulation. *Amer. J. Med.* 77(3A):2–8, 1984.

Fields, H. L., and Levine, J. D. Biology of placebo analgesia. *Amer. J. Med.* 70:745–746, 1981.

Fisher, P., and Ward, A. Complementary medicine in Europe. *Brit. Med. J.* 309:107–110, 1994.

Fitzgerald, F. S. Quoted in Lefton, Chronic disease and applied sociology.

Flexner, A. *Medical education in the United States and Canada.* New York: Carnegie Foundation, 1910.

Fordtran, J. S. Placebos, antacids, and cimetidine for duodenal ulcer. *New Eng. J. Med.* 298:1081–1083, 1978.

Frank, A. *At the will of the body: reflections on illness.* Boston: Houghton Mifflin, 1991.

————. *The wounded storyteller: body, illness and ethics.* Chicago: University of Chicago Press, 1995.

Frank, J. D. *Persuasion and healing.* New York: Schocken, 1970, p. 3.

Freidson, E. Disability as social deviance. In *Medical men and their work*, ed. E. Freidson and J. Lorber. Chicago: Aldine-Atherton, 1972, p. 330.

Fried, C. *Contract as promise: a theory of contractual obligation.* Cambridge: Harvard University Press, 1981.

Gallagher, E. J., Viscoli, C. M., and Horwitz, R. I. The relationship of treatment adherence to the risks of death after myocardial infarction in women. *JAMA* 207:742–744, 1993.

Gevitz, N. Christian Science healing and the health of children. *Perspectives Biol. Med.* 34:421–438, 1991.

Glymour, C., and Stalker, D. Engineers, cranks, physicians, magicians. *New Eng. J. Med.* 308:960–964, 1983.

Goddard, H. H. The effect of mind on body as evidenced by faith cures. *Amer. J. Psycho.* 10 (1894). Quoted in James, *Varieties of religious experience*, p. 95.

Good, B. *Medicine, rationality and experience: an anthropological perspective.* Cambridge: Cambridge University Press, 1994.

Goodwin, J. S., Goodwin, J. M., and Vogel, A. V. Knowledge and use of placebos by house officers and nurses. *Ann. Intern. Med.* 91:106–110, 1979.

Gordon, J. S. Why patients choose alternative medicine. *Internist* 35:6–9, 1994.

Gowers, W. *Manual of disease of the nervous system.* 1886.

Gracely, R. H., Dubner, R., Deeter, W. R., et al. Clinicians' expectations influence placebo analgesia. *Lancet* 1:43, 1985.

Green, D. M. Pre-existing conditions, placebo reactions and "side effects." *Ann. Intern. Med.* 60:255–265, 1964.

Grunbaum, A. The placebo concept. *Behav. Res. Therapy* 19:157–167, 1981.

Gudjonsson, B., and Spiro, H. M. Response to placebos in ulcer disease. *Amer. J. Med.* 65:399–402, 1978.

Gutheil, T. G., and Havens, L. L. The therapeutic alliance: contemporary meanings and confusions. *Int. Rev. Psycho. Anal.* 6:467–479, 1979.

Hahn, R. A. *Sickness and healing: an anthropological perspective.* New Haven: Yale University Press, 1995.

Hahn, R. A., and Kleinman, A. Biomedical practice and anthropological theory. *Ann. Rev. Anthropol.* 12:305–333, 1983.

Harner, M. *Way of the shaman: a guide to power and healing.* San Francisco: Harper and Row, 1980.

Harrington, A. Cracking open the black box of placebos. *Harvard Medical Alumni Bull.* 68:34–40, 1995 (Winter).

Harrington, A., ed. *The placebo effect*. Cambridge: Harvard University Press, 1997.

Hart, F. D. Pain as an old friend. Brit. Med. J. 1:1405–1407, 1979.

Hart, J. T., and Dieppe, P. Caring effects. *Lancet* 347:1606–1608, 1996.

Havens, L. L. Explorations in the uses of language in psychotherapy: simple empathic statements. *Psychiatry* 41:336–344, 1978.

Hawkins, A. H. *Reconstructing illness: studies in pathography*. West Lafayette, Ind.: Purdue University Press, 1993.

Hawkins v. McGee. Supreme Court of New Hampshire, 1929. Cited in *Contracts*, ed. J. R. Dawson, W. B. Harvey, and S. D. Henderson. Mineola, N.Y.: Foundation Press, 1982, pp. 1–4.

Heisenberg, W. *Physics and beyond: encounters and conversation*. New York: Harper, 1972, p. 63.

Held, V. *Feminist morality transforming culture, society, and politics*. Chicago: University of Chicago Press, 1993.

Helms, J. M. Acupuncture for the management of primary dysmenorrhea. *Obstet. Gynec.* 69:51–56, 1987.

Henderson, L. J. Physician and patient as a social system. *New Eng. J. Med.* 212:819–823, 1935.

Hippocrates. Precepts V.I. In *Hippocrates*, trans. W. H. S. Jones. New York: G. P. Putnam's Sons, 1923, p. 319.

Homer. *The Iliad*. Trans. Robert Fitzgerald. New York: Anchor, 1975.

Horwitz, R. I., and Horwitz, S. M. Adherence to treatment and health outcomes. *Arch. Intern. Med.* 153:1863–1868, 1993.

Horwitz, R. I., Viscoli, C. M., Berkham, L., et al. Treatment adherence and risk of death after a myocardial infarction. *Lancet* 336:542–545, 1993.

Houston, W. R. The doctor himself as a therapeutic agent. *Ann. Intern. Med.* 11:1416–1425, 1938.

Howell, J. D. The X-ray image: meaning, gender and power. In *Technology in the hospital: transforming patient care in the early twentieth century*. Baltimore, Md.: Johns Hopkins University Press, 1995.

Hufford, D. J. Epistemologies in religious healing. *J. Med. Phil.* 18:175–194, 1993.

Illich, I. *Medical nemesis*. London: Calder and Boyars, 1975, pp. 31–66. (New edition, 1996.)

Ingelfinger, F. J. Arrogance. *New Eng. J. Med.* 303:1507–1511, 1980.

International Association for the Study of Pain (IASP) Subcommittee on Taxonomy Pain Terms. *Pain* 6:249–252, 1979.

Jackson, S. W. L. The listening healer in the history of psychological healing. *Amer. J. Psychiatry* 149:1623–1632, 1992.

Jacobs, H. R. Intuition: the welcome stranger. *Perspectives Biol. Med.* 24:457–466, 1981.

Jacobs, J. J. Unproven alternative methods of cancer treatment. In DeVita, Hellman, and Rosenberg, *Principles and practices of oncology*, pp. 2993–3001.

James, W. *The principles of psychology*, vol. 1. New York: Dover, 1980.

————. *The varieties of religious experience*. New York: Modern Library, 1902.

Jensen, M. D., and Karoly, P. Motivation and expectation factors in symptom perception: a laboratory study of the placebo-effect. *Psychosom. Med.* 33:144–152, 1991.

Jewson, N. D. The disappearance of the sick-man from medical cosmology, 1770–1870. *Sociology* 10:225–244, 1976.

Johnson, A. G. Surgery as a placebo. *Lancet* 334:1140–1142, 1994.

Jones, A. H. Literature in medicine: narrative of mental illness. *Lancet* 350:359–361, 1997.

Jones, J. K. Do over-the-counter drugs act mainly as placebos? Yes. In *Controversies in therapeutics*, ed. L. Lasagna. Philadelphia: Saunders, 1980, pp. 26–32.

Jospe, M. *The placebo effect*. Lexington, Mass.: D. C. Heath, 1978.

Joyce, C. R. B. Placebo and complementary medicine. *Lancet* 344:1279–1281, 1994.

Jung, C. *Answer to Job*. New York: Meridian, 1962, p. 14.

————. *Modern man in search of a soul*. New York: Harcourt, Brace, Jovanovich, 1922, p. 225.

Jurcich v. General Motors Corp. 539 S.W. 2d 595 (Mo. App. 1976).

Kahn, S. The anatomy of Norman Cousins's illness. *Mt. Sinai J. Med.* 48:305–314, 1981.

Kandell, E. R., and Schwartz, S. H. Molecular biology of learning. *Science* 218:433–443, 1982.

Kapp, U. B. Placebo therapy and the law: prescribe with care. *Amer. J. L. Med.* 8:371, 1982.

Katz, J. *The silent world of doctor and patient*. New York: Free Press, 1984.

Kaunitz, P. the favorable prognosis. *Conn. Med.* 49:542, 1985.

Kiecolt-Glaser, J. K., Maruch, P. T., Malarkey, W. B., et al. Slowing of wound healing by psychological stress. *Lancet* 346:1194–1196, 1995.

King, L. S. The Flexner report of 1910. *JAMA* 251:1079–1086, 1984.

Kirsch, I. Response expectancy as a determinant of experience and behavior. *American Psychologist* 40:1189–1202, 1985.

Kleijnen, J., Decrean, J. M., Van Everdingen, J., et al. Placebo effect in double-blind clinical trials: a review of interactions with medications. *Lancet* 344:1347–1349, 1994.

Kleinman, A. Neurasthenia and depression. *Culture, Medicine and Psychiatry* 6:117–190, 1982.

————. *Patients and healers in the context of culture.* Berkeley: University of California Press, 1980, p. 361.

Kleinman, A., Eisenberg, L., and Good, B. Culture, illness, and care: clinical lessons from anthropologic and cross-cultural research. *Ann. Intern. Med.* 88:251–258, 1978.

Kleinman, A., and Sung, L. Why do indigenous practitioners successfully heal? *Soc. Sci. Med.* 13B:7–26, 1976.

Klopfer, B. Psychological variables in human cancer. *J. Projective Techniques* 21:331–340, 1957.

Konotey-Ahulu, F. Personal interview. *Brit. Med. J.* 1:1595, 1977.

Konvitz, M. R. Loyalty. In *Dictionary of the history of ideas*, vol. 3, ed. R. P. Wiener. New York: Scribner, 1973, pp. 108–116.

Krakauer, E. L. Attending to dying. In Spiro, Curnen, and Wandel, *Facing death.*

Kronenberg, F., Mallory, B., and Downey, J. A. Rehabilitation medicine and alternative therapy: new words, old practices. *Arch. Phys. Med. Rehabil.* 75:928–929, 1994.

Krumbhaar, E. B. *A history of medicine.* New York: Knopf, 1941.

Krystal, H. Self-representation and the capacity for self-care. *Annual of Psychoanalysis* 6:209–246, 1977.

Kussler, W. J., Blanc, P., and Greenblatt, R. The use of medicinal herbs by human immunovirus infected patients. *Arch. Intern. Med.* 151:2209–2288, 1991.

Lakoff, G., and Johnson, M. Conceptual metaphor in everyday language. *J. Philosophy* 77:453–486, 1980.

Landy, D., ed. *Culture, disease and healing.* New York: Macmillan, 1977.

Lants, P. M., and Reding, D. Cancer: beliefs and attitudes of Latinos. *JAMA* 272:31–32, 1994.

Laporte, J. R., and Figueras, A. Placebo effects in psychiatry. *Lancet* 344:1206–1209, 1994.

Lasagna, L., Laties, V. G., and Dohan, J. L. Further studies on the "pharmacology" of placebo administration. *J. Clin. Invest.* 37:533–537, 1958.

Lefton, M. Chronic disease and applied sociology: an essay in personalized sociology. *Sociological Inquiry* 54:466–476, 1984.

Lerner, M. Healing. In Moyers, *Healing and the mind.*

————. *New York Times Magazine*, October 2, 1994, p. 63 ff.

Leslie, A. Ethics and practice of placebo therapy. *Amer. J. Med.* 16:854–862, 1954.

————. Letter. *Ann. Intern. Med.* 97:781, 1982.

Letters. *New Eng. J. Med.* 332:60–62, 1995.

Levenstein, S. Wellness, health, Antonovsky. *Advances: The Journal of Mind Body Health* 10:26–29, 1994.

Lewin, K. *Field theory in social science.* New York: Harper, 1964.

Lewis, C. S. *The problem of pain.* New York: Macmillan, 1943.

Lewith, G. T., and Machin, D. On the evaluation of the clinical effects of acupuncture. *Pain* 16:111–127, 1983.

Li, Y., Tougas, G., Chiverton, S. G., et al. The effect of acupuncture on gastrointestinal function and disorder. *Amer. J. Gastroenterol.* 84:1372–1389, 1992.

Licinio, J., Gold, P. W., and Wong, M.-L. A molecular mechanism for stress induced alterations in susceptibility to disease. *Lancet* 346:104–106, 1995.

Lin, K. M. Hwa-Byung: a Korean cultural syndrome? *Amer. J. Psychiatry* 140:105–107, 1983.

Lipkin, M. Suggestion and healing. *Perspectives Biol. Med.* 28:121–126, 1984.

Lipkin, M., McDevitt, E., Schwartz, S., et al. On the effects of suggestion in the treatment of vasospastic disorders of the extremities. *Psychosom Med.* 7:152–157, 1945.

Lipman, J. L., Miller, B. E., Mayas, K. S., et al. Peak beta-endorphin concentrations in cerebral spinal fluid: reduced in chronic pain patients and increased during the placebo response. *Psychopharmacology* 102:112–116, 1990.

Lipowski, Z. S. Psychosocial aspects of disease. *Ann. Intern. Med.* 71:1197–1206, 1969.

———. Somatization: the concept and its clinical application. *Amer. J. Psychiatry* 14:1358–1368, 1988.

Littlewood, R. From disease to illness and back again. *Lancet* 337:1013–1016, 1991.

Liu Yanchi. *Essential book of traditional Chinese medicine.* Vol. 2. New York: Columbia University Press, 1988.

Lock, M. *East Asian medicine in urban Japan.* Berkeley, University of California Press, 1980.

Loesser, J. D. What is chronic pain? *Theoretical Medicine* 12:247–270, 1991.

Lown, B. *The lost art of healing.* Boston: Houghton Mifflin, 1997.

———. Personal communication. June 6, 1985.

———. Verbal conditioning of angina pectoris during exercise testing. *Amer. J. Cardiol.* 40:630–634, 1977.

MacDonald, A. J., Peden, N. R., Hayton, R., et al. Symptom relief and the placebo effect in the trial of an antipeptic drug. *Gut* 22:323–336, 1981.

Margulis, J. The concept of disease. *J. Med. Phil.* 1:238–255, 1976.

Martin, S. C. The only truly scientific method of healing: chiropractic and medical science, 1895–1990. *Isis* 5:206–227, 1994.

Matthews, D. A., Suchman, A. L., and Branch, W. T. Making "connexions": enhancing the therapeutic potential of patient-clinician relationships. *Ann. Intern. Med.* 118:973–977, 1993.

May, W. F. *The physician's covenant: images of the healer's medical ethics.* Philadelphia: Westminster, 1983.

McClenon, J. The experiential foundations of shamanic healing. *J. Med. Phil.* 18:107–127, 1993.

McLuhan, M. *Understanding media.* New York: McGraw-Hill, 1964.

McWhinney, I. R., Epstein, R. M., and Freeman, T. R. Rethinking somatization. *Ann. Intern. Med.* 126:747–750, 1997.

Mead, M. Concept of culture and the psychosomatic approach. *Psychiatry* 10:57–76, 1947.

Medawar, P. S. *Induction and intuition in scientific thought.* Philadelphia: American Philosophical Society, 1969, p. 29.

Melzach, R. Pain: past, present and future. *Canadian J. of Experimental Psychology* 47:615–629, 1993.

———. *The puzzle of pain.* New York: Basic, 1973.

Mendelson, G., Selwood, T. S., Kranz, H., et al. Acupuncture treatment of chronic low back pain. *Amer. J. Med.* 74:49–55, 1983.

Mermann, A. C. The whole physician divided in three parts. *Pharos* 57:7–10, 1994.

Meyer, E. A., and Gebhart, G. F. Basic and clinical aspects of visceral hyperalgesia. *Gastroenterology* 107:271–293, 1994.

Meyers, S., and Janowitz, H. D. The "natural history" of Crohn's disease: an analytic review of the placebo lesson. *Gastroenterology* 87:1189–1192, 1984.

Miller, N. E. Behavioral medicine: symbiosis between laboratory and clinic. *Ann. Rev. Psycho.* 34:1–31, 1983.

Moerman, D. E. Anthropology of symbolic healing. *Current Anthropol.* 20:59–80, 1979.

———. Physiology and symbols: the anthropological implications of the placebo effect. In *The anthropology of medicine,* ed. L. Romanucci-Ross, D. E. Moerman, and L. R. Tancredi. New York: Praeger, 1983.

Montague, W. P. Quoted in H. H. Titus and M. S. Smith, *Living issues in philosophy.* 6th ed. New York: Van Nostrand, 1974, p. 242.

Montgomery, G., and Kirsch, I. Classical conditioning and the placebo effect. *Pain* 72:107–113, 1997.

Morris, D. *The culture of pain.* Berkeley: University of California Press, 1993.

———. What we make of pain. *Wilson Quarterly* 18:8–26, 1994.

Morris, H. Suggestion in the treatment of disease. *Brit. Med. J.* 1:1457–1466, 1910.

Morrison, P. Turkey: Placebo effect. *Lancet* 337:1213–1214, 1991.

Moyers, B. *Healing and the mind.* New York, Doubleday, 1995.

Murray, R. H., and Rubel, A. J. Physicians and healers—unwitting partners in healthcare. *New Eng. J. Med.* 326:61–64, 1992.

National Institutes of Health (NIH) Technology Assessment Panel. Integration of behavioral and relaxation approaches in the treatment of chronic pain and insomnia. *JAMA* 267:313–318, 1996.

Newton, L. The healing of the person. *Conn. Med.* 41:641–646, 1977.

Nie, J.-B. The physician as general. *JAMA* 276:1099, 1996.

O'Neill, A. Danger and safety in medicine. *Soc. Sci. Med.* 38:497–507, 1994.

Ong., W. J. *Interfaces of the word.* Ithaca, N.Y.: Cornell University Press, 1977, chap. 5.

Owen, D. Medicine, morality, and the market. *Lancet* 2:30–31, 1984.

Ozick, C. Puttermesser. In *Levitation: five fictions.* New York: Knopf, 1982.

Packer, M. A placebo effect in heart failure. *Amer. Heart J.* 120:1579–1582, 1990.

Pangle, T. L. *The laws of Plato.* New York: Basic Books, 1980.

Papac, R. J. Spontaneous regression of cancer. *Cancer Treatment Reviews* 22:395–423, 1996.

Parker, J. O. Efficacy of nitroglycerine patches: fact or fancy? *Ann. Intern. Med.* 102:548–549, 1985.

Payer, Lynn. *Medicine and culture.* New York: Penguin, 1988.

Pearce, J. M. The placebo enigma. *Quarterly J. Med.* 88:215–220, 1995.

Peck, C., and Coleman, G. Implications of placebo therapy for clinical research and practice in pain management. *Theoretical Med.* 12:247–270, 1991.

Peek, M. I. Traditional African medicine. *Pharos.* Spring: 24–29, 1995.

Perry, S., and Fishman, B. Depression and HIV—how does one affect the other? *JAMA* 270:2609–2610, 1993.

Phillips, D., and Smith, D. G. Postponement of death until symbolically meaning occasions. *JAMA* 263:1947–1951, 1990.

Phillips, D. D., Ruth, T., and Wagner, L. M. Psychology and survival. *Lancet* 342:1142–1145, 1993.

Phillips, W. R. Patients, pills, and professionals: the ethics of placebo therapy. *Pharos* 44:21–25, 1981.

Plato. *The republic.* New York: Scribner's Sons, 1928, book 3, p. 121.

Polanyi, M. Life's irreducible structures. In *Knowing and being: essays,* ed. Marjorie Grene. Chicago: University of Chicago Press, 1969.

Prince, R. H. Psychotherapy as the manipulation of endogenous healing mechanisms: a transcultural survey. *Trans-cultural Psychiatry Research Review* 13:115–133, 1976.

Prioleau, L., Murdock, M., and Brody, N. An analysis of psychotherapy versus placebo studies. *Behavior Brain Sci.* 6:275–285, 1983.

Rawls, J. *A theory of justice.* Cambridge: Harvard University Press, Belknap, 1971.

Risjord, M. Relativism and the social scientific study of medicine. *J. Med. Phil.* 18:195–212, 1993.

Roethlisberger, F. J., and Dickson, W. J. *Management and the workers.* Cambridge: Harvard University Press, 1939.

Rogers, S. L. *The shaman, his symbols and his healing power.* Springfield, Ill.: Thomas, 1982.

Rorty, R. *Philosophy and the mirror of nature.* Princeton, N.J.: Princeton University Press, 1979, p. 38.

Rose, S. The rise of neurogenetic determinism. *Nature* 373:380–382, 1995.

Rosen, D. H. Inborn basis for the healing doctor-patient relationship. *Pharos,* Fall: 17–22, 1992.

Rothman, K. J., and Michels, K. B. The continuing unethical use of placebo controls. *New Eng. J. Med.* 331:394–398, 1994.

Royce, J. *The philosophy of loyalty.* New York: Macmillan, 1928.

Ruberman, W., Weinblatt, E., Goldberg, J. D., et al. Psychosocial influences on mortality after myocardial infarction. *New Eng. J. Med.* 311:552–559, 1984.

Ruderman, F. A. A placebo for the doctor. *Commentary,* May: 54–60, 1980.

Rueschemeyer, D. Doctors and lawyers: a comment on the theory of the profession. In *Medical men and their work,* ed. E. Freidson, and J. Lorber. Chicago: Aldine-Atherton, 1972.

Russell, B. *Mysticism and logic.* Garden City, N.Y.: Doubleday, 1957.

———. *Religion and science.* London: Oxford University Press, 1935, pp. 8, 178.

Sachar, D. Placebo-controlled clinical trials in gastroenterology. *Amer. J. Gastroenterol.* 79:913–917, 1984.

Sampson, R. Healing in the treatment of modern medicine. *Somatics* 1978:8–14.

Sandler, R. S., Drossman, D. A., Nathan, H. D., et al. Symptom complaints and health care seeking behavior in subjects with bowel dysfunction. *Gastroenterology* 87:314–318, 1984.

Sarles, H., Camatte, R., and Sahel, J. A study of the variation in the response regarding duodenal ulcer when treated with placebo by different investigators. *Digestion* 16:289–292, 1997.

Scarry, E. *The body in pain.* New York: Oxford University Press, 1985.

Schmidt, S. A. When you come into my room. *JAMA* 276:512, 1996.

Schonauer, K. *Semiotic foundations of drug therapy: the placebo problem in a new perspective.* Berlin: Morton de Gruyter, 1994.

Shalev, M. *Esau.* New York: HarperCollins, 1991.

Shall I please? *Lancet* 2:1465–1466, 1983.

Shapiro, A. K. A contribution to a history of the placebo effect. *Behavioral Science* 5:109–135, 1960.

———. Factors contributing to the placebo effect. *Amer. J. Psychiatry* 18:73–88, 1964.

———. The placebo response. In *Modern perspectives in world psychiatry*, vol. 2, ed. J. G. Howells. Edinburgh: Oliver and Budy, 1971.

Shekelle, P. G., Adams, A. H., Chassin, M. R., et al. Spinal manipulation of low back pain. *Ann. Intern. Med.* 117:590–598, 1992.

Shore, M. F., and Beigel, A. The challenges posed by managed behavioral health care. *New Eng. J. Med.* 334:116–118, 1996.

Shryock, R. H. The history of quantification in medical science. *Isis* 52:215–237, 1961.

Siegler, M. Clinical illness: the limits of autonomy. *Hastings Center Report* 7:12–15, 1977.

Silber, T. J. Placebo therapy: the ethical dimension. *JAMA* 242:245–246, 1979.

Simmons, B. Problems in deceptive medical procedures: an ethical and legal analysis of the administration of placebos. *J. Med. Ethics* 4:172–181, 1978.

Simonton, O., Matthews-Simonton, S., and Creighton, J. *Getting well again*. Los Angeles: Tarcher, 1978.

Simpson, J. The stigmata: pathology or miracle? *Brit. Med. J.* 289:1746–1748, 1984.

Sims, A. *Symptoms in the mind*. 2d ed. London: Saunders, 1995.

Singer, D. L., and Hurwitz, D. Long-term experience with sulfonylureas and placebo. *New Eng. J. Med.* 277:450–456, 1967.

Sivin, N. *Traditional medicine in contemporary China*. Ann Arbor: Center for Chinese Studies, University of Michigan, 1987.

Skovlund, E. Should we tell trial patients that they might receive a placebo? *Lancet* 337:1041, 1991.

Skrabanek, P. Acupuncture and the age of unreason. *Lancet* 1:1169–1171, 1984.

Skrabanek, P., and McCormick, J. *Follies and fallacies in medicine*. Glasgow: Terragon Press, 1989.

Smith, J. C. *Royce's social infinite: the community of interpretation*. Hamden, Conn.: Anchor, 1969.

Smith, L. F. Folk medical beliefs and their implications for care of patients. *Ann. Intern. Med.* 81:82–96, 1974.

Smith, M. *The white lie*. Unpublished manuscript.

Sontag, S. *AIDS and its metaphors*. New York: Farrar, Straus and Giroux, 1989.

Spicker, S. F. Terra firma and infirma species. J. Med. Phil. 1:104–135, 1976.

Spiegel, D. Psychological distress and disease course for women with breast cancer: one answer, many questions. J. Nat. Cancer Inst. 88:629–631, 1996.

Spiegel, D., Bloom, J. R., Kraemer, H. C., et al. Effectiveness of psychosocial treatment on survival of patients with metastatic breast cancer. Lancet 2:888–891, 1989.

Spiro, H. M. Clinical gastroenterology. 4th ed. New York: Miller, 1993. (1st ed., 1970.)

——. Mammon and medicine: the rewards of clinical trials. JAMA 255:1174–1175, 1980.

Spiro, H., Curnen, M., Peschel, E., St. James, D. Empathy and the practice of medicine. New Haven: Yale University Press, 1993.

Spiro, H. M., Curnen, M. C., and Wandel, L. P., eds. Facing death: where culture, religion, and medicine meet. New Haven: Yale University Press, 1996.

Starck, D. L. Enhancing hope in the chronically ill. Humane Medicine 9:103–130, 1993.

Starr, P. The social transformation of American medicine. New York: Basic Books, 1982.

Stein, C. The control of pain in peripheral tissues by opioids. New Eng. J. Med. 332:1685–1690, 1995.

Stoeckle, J. D., Zola, I. K., and Davidson, G. E. The quantity and significance of psychosocial distress in medical patients. J. Chr. Dis. 17:959–970, 1964.

Subbarayappa, B. V. Siddha medicine: an overview. Lancet 350:1841–1844, 1997.

Suchman, A. L. A model of empathic communication in a medical interview. JAMA 277:678–682, 1997.

Suchman, A. L., and Ader, R. Classic conditioning and placebo effects in crossover studies. Clin. Pharmacol. Ther. 52:372–377, 1992.

Sullivan, M. D. Placebo controls and epistemic control in orthodox medicine. J. Med. Phil. 18:213–231, 1993.

Swan, R. Faith-healing, Christian Science, and the medical care of children. New Eng. J. Med. 209:1639–1641, 1983.

Szasz, T. Diagnoses are not diseases. Lancet 338:1574–1576, 1991.

Talbot, N. A. The position of the Christian Science church. New Eng. J. Med. 209:1641–1644, 1983.

Tatara, K. On putting life first. Lancet 346:327–328, 1995.

Taylor, C. E. Positive illusions: creative self-deception and the healthy mind. New York: Basic Books, 1989.

Ter Reit, G., Kleijnen, J., and Knipschild, P. Acupuncture and chronic pain: a criteria based meta-analysis. *J. Clin. Epidemiol.* 43:1191–1199, 1990.

Tessman, I., and Tessman, J. Mind and body. (Book review.) *Science* 276:369–370, 1997.

Thomasma, D. C. Beyond medical paternalism and patient autonomy: a model of physician conscience for the physician-patient relationship. *Ann. Intern. Med.* 98:243–248, 1983.

———. Limitations of the autonomy model for the doctor-patient relationship, *Pharos* 46:2–5, 1983.

Tross, S., Herndon, J., Krazun, A., et al. Psychological symptoms and disease free and overall survival in women with stage II breast cancer. *J. Nat. Cancer Inst.* 88:661–667, 1996.

Tseng, W. S. The nature of somatic complaints among psychiatric patients: the Chinese case. *Comp. Psychiatry* 16:237–245, 1945.

Turner, J. A., Deo, R. A., Loeser, J. D., et al. The importance of placebo effects in pain treatment and research. *JAMA* 271:1609–1614, 1994.

Veatch, R. M. *A theory of medical ethics.* New York: Basic Books, 1981.

Viseltear, A. J. Milton C. Winternitz and the Yale Institute of Human Relations: a brief chapter in the history of social medicine. *Yale J. Biol. Med.* 57:869–889, 1984.

Wall, P. D. The placebo effect: an unpopular topic. *Pain* 51:1–3, 1992.

Ward, P. S. The medical brothers Cabot: of truth and consequence. *Harvard Med. Alumni Bull.* 56:30–39, 1982.

Warner, J. H. *The therapeutic perspective.* Cambridge: Harvard University Press, 1986.

Warshafsky, S., Kamer, R. S., and Sivak, S. L. Effect of garlic on total serum cholesterol: a meta-analysis. *Ann. Intern. Med.* 119:599–605, 1993.

Weil, A. *Spontaneous healing: how to discover and enhance your body's natural ability to heal itself.* New York: Knopf, 1995.

Weiss, E., and English, O. S. *Psychosomatic medicine.* Philadelphia: Saunders, 1943.

Wellek, R. Romanticism in literature. In *Dictionary of the history of ideas,* vol. 2, ed. R. P. Wiener. New York: Scribner, 1973, pp. 187–198.

White, L. Technical assessment from the stance of a medical historian. *Amer. Hist. Rev.* 79:1–13, 1974.

White, L., Tursky, B., and Schwartz, G. *Placebo: theory, research, and mechanisms.* New York: Guilford Press, 1985.

Williams, R. B. The role of the brain in physical disease. *JAMA* 263:197–198, 1990.

Winslow, G. R. From loyalty to advocacy: a new metaphor for nursing. *Hastings Center Report,* June: 32–39, 1984.

Winters, C., Artnak, E. J., Benjamin, S. B., et al. Esophageal bouginage in symptomatic patients with the nutcracker esophagus. *JAMA* 252:363–366, 1984.

Wittgenstein, L. The blue and brown books. New York: Harper and Row, 1965, p. 18.

Wolf, S. The pharmacology of placebos. *Pharmacologic Rev.* 11:689–704, 1959.

Wolf, S., and Wolff, H. *Human gastric function.* London: Oxford University Press, 1947.

Wolff, B. B. Ethnocultural factors influencing pain and illness behavior. *Clin. J. Pain* 1:23–80, 1985.

Wolff, B. B., and Langley, F. Culture and pain. *Amer. Anthropol.* 70:494–501, 1968.

Wolff, H. G., DuBois, F., and Gold, H. Cornell conferences on therapy: use of placebos in therapy. *New York J. Med.* 46:1718–1727, 1946.

Wolpe, P. R. The maintenance of professional authority: acupuncture and the American physician. *Social Problems* 32:409–424, 1985.

Yuan, Y. L., Tougas, G., Chiverton, S., et al. The effect of acupuncture on gastrointestinal function and disorders. *Amer. J. Gastroenterol.* 87:1372–1381, 1992.

Zinsser, H. *As I remember him: the biography of R.S.* Boston: Little, Brown, 1941, pp. 140–141.

Other References

The references included here are for scholars who want to trace the sources of various statements not otherwise attributed. The statements are sometimes quoted and sometimes in indirect discourse. The sources are listed here by chapter in the order in which they are pertinent.

chapter two
The Placebo Drama

Roethlisberger, F. J., and Dickson, W. J. *Management and the workers*. Cambridge: Harvard University Press, 1939.

Gudjonsson, B., and Spiro, H. M. Response to placebos in ulcer disease. *Amer. J. Med.* 65:399–402, 1978.

Blum, A. L. Is placebo the ideal anti-ulcer drug? In *Peptic ulcer disease*, ed. G. Bianchig and K. D. Bardhan. New York: Raven Press, 1982, pp. 57–61.

MacDonald, A. J., Peden, N. R., Hayton, R., et al. Symptom relief and the placebo effect in the trial of an anti-peptic drug. *Gut* 21:323–326, 1980.

Littman, A., Welch, R., Fruin, R. C., et al. Control trials of aluminum hydroxide gels for peptic ulcer. *Gastroenterology* 73:6–10, 1977.

Sarles, H., Camatte, R., and Sahel, J. A study of the variations and the response regarding duodenal ulcers when treated with placebo by different investigators. *Digestion* 16:289–292, 1977.

Peterson, W. L., and Elashoff, J. Placebos in clinical trials of duodenal ulcer: the end of an ear? *Gastroenterology* 79:585–588, 1980.

Meyers, S., and Janowitz, H. D. The "natural history" of Crohn's disease: an analytic review of the placebo lesson. *Gastroenterology* 87:1189–1192, 1984.

Wolff, H. G., DuBois, F., and Gold, H. Cornell conferences on therapy: uses of placebo in therapy. *New York J. Med.* 46:718–727, 1946.

Bond, M. *Pain: its nature, analysis and treatment*. New York: Churchill Livingstone, 1979, p. 135.

Brody, H. The lie that heals: the ethics of giving placebos. *Ann. Intern. Med.* 97:112–118, 1982.

chapter three
The Physician

Stoeckle, J. D., Zola, I. K., and Davidson, G. E. The quantity and significance of psychological distress in medical patients. *J. Chr. Dis.* 17:959–970, 1964.

chapter four
Pills and Procedures

Spiro, H. M. Is milk so bad for the peptic ulcer patient? *J. Clin. Gastroenterol.* 3:219–220, 1981.

chapter five
The Patient and the Disease

Cobb, L. A., Thomas, G. I., Dillard, D. H., et al. An evaluation of internal mammary-artery ligation by a double-blind technique. *New Eng. J. Med.* 260:1115–1118, 1959.

Benson, H., and McCallie, D. P. Angina pectoris and the placebo effect. *New Eng. J. Med.* 300:1424–1429, 1979.

Winters, C., Artnak, E. J., Benjamin, S. B., et al. Esophageal bouginage in symptomatic patients with the nutcracker esophagus. *JAMA* 252:363–366, 1984.

Riddell, R. H., Goldman, H., Ransohoff, D. F., et al. Dysplasia in inflammatory bowel disease. *Human Path.* 14:931–968, 1983.

chapter six
What Placebos Can Do

Wolf, S. The pharmacology of placebos. *Pharmacologic. Rev.* 11:689–704, 1959.

Green, D. M. Preexisting conditions, placebo reactions, and "side-effects." *Ann. Intern. Med.* 60:255–265, 1964.

Everson, T. C., and Cole, W. H. *Spontaneous regression of cancer.* Philadelphia: Saunders, 1966, p. 4.

Wolf, S., and Wolff, H. *Human gastric function.* London: Oxford University Press, 1947.

Singer, D. L., and Herwitz, D. Long-term experience with sulfonylureas and placebos. *New Eng. J. Med.* 277:450–456, 1967.

Frost, F. A., Jessen, B., and Sigaard-Anderson, J. A control, double-blind comparison of mepivacaine injection versus saline injection for myofascial pain. *Lancet* 1:499–500, 1980.

Park, L. C., and Covi, L. Nonblind placebo trial: an exploration of neurotic outpatients' responses to placebo when its inert content is disclosed. *Arch. J. Psychiatry.* 12:336–345, 1965.

Blackwell, B., Bloomfield, S. S., and Buncher, C. R. Demonstration to medical students of placebo responses and non-drug factors. *Lancet* 1:1279–1282, 1972.

chapter seven
Patients and Pain

Wolff, B. B. Ethnocultural factors influencing pain and illness behavior. *Clin. J. Pain* 1:23–80, 1985.

Zborowski, M. Cultural components and responses to pain. *J. Soc. Issues* 8:16–30, 1952.

chapter nine
Objections to Placebos

Leslie, A. Ethics and practice of placebo therapy. *Am. J. Med.* 16:854–862, 1954.

Leslie, A. Letter. *Ann. Intern. Med.* 97:781, 1982.

Silber, T. J. Placebo therapy: the ethical dimension. *JAMA* 242:245–246, 1979.

Adler, H. M., and Hammett, V. O. The doctor-patient relationship revisited: analysis of the placebo effect. *Ann. Intern. Med.* 78:595–598, 1975.

chapter ten
Alternative Medicine

Goddard, H. H. The effect of mind on body as evidenced by faith cures. *Amer. J. Psycho.* 10 (1894). Quoted in W. James, *The varieties of religious experience.* New York: Modern Library, 1902, p. 95.

Davies, G. The hands of the healer: has faith a place? *J. Med. Ethics* 6:185–189, 1980.

chapter eleven
Placebos, Alternative Medicine, and Healing

Landy, D., ed. *Culture, disease and healing.* New York: Macmillan, 1977.

Moerman, D. E. Anthropology of symbolic healing. *Current Anthropol.* 20:59–80, 1979.

Prince, R. H. Psychotherapy as the manipulation of endogenous healing mechanisms: a transcultural survey. *Transcultural Psychiatry Research Review* 13:115–133, 1976.

Homer. *The iliad*. Trans. Robert Fitzgerald. New York: Anchor, 1974.

Toynbee, A. J. *A study of history*. London: Oxford University Press, 1948.

Wellek, R. Romanticism in literature. In *Dictionary of the history of ideas*, vol. 2, ed. R. P. Wiener. New York: Scribner, 1973, pp. 187–198.

Index

Cousins, Norman, 4–5, 103–108, 119, 214, 237

Covenant, 220–221

Culture: alternative medicine and, 134; in construction of disease, 231, 255n1; effects of, on reactions to disease/pain, 96, 154–163; and medicine, 185, 192–193; and following medical advice, 142; personalistic versus naturalistic systems, 163–164

Culture of Pain (Morris), 92–93

Cure: versus care, 2–3, 8; versus relief of symptoms, 13

Dance therapy, 180

Davidoff, Leo, 113–114

Deception. *See* Truth-telling

Deduction and science, 193–194

Delayed gastric emptying, 44

Depression, 56; and AIDS, 147; and chronic pain, 94; and healing in non-Western cultures, 155–156, 159; physical effects of, 205; and placebos, 162–163; theories on causes of, 200, 215, 250n3

Diabetes, 79–80

Diagnostic tests: as placebos, 25, 41, 152; reliance on, in mainstream medicine, 61–65, 248n4

Dicks, Russell, 115–116

Dietary supplements, 39, 153

Disease: culture in construction of, 231, 255n1; defining, 51–52, 53, 250n1; as distinct from illness, x, 2, 8, 51, 52; placebos and effect on, 83–86; views of modern medicine on, 59–60

Disorder, definition of, 51, 53

Distrust of mainstream medicine, 143

Doctors, Patients, and Placebos (Spiro), x

Double-blind trials, 14–15

Drugs: dependency on, and acupuncture, 172; pain relief, 101

Dunbar, Flanders, 210

Dyspepsia, 294n1

Edelstein, Ludwig, 219

Education, medical, 187–192, 195–196

Einstein, Albert, 192

Eisenberg, David, 84, 139

Eisenberg, Leon, 52

Emerson, Ralph Waldo, 68

Emmanuel Movement, 167–168

Emotional disorders, and non-Western cultures, 156, 159, 171

Emotions: effect on illness and disease, 32, 54–55, 66–67, 160–163, 201–205, 234–236; healing and positive, 106–107; modern medicine and attitudes toward, 56–57; and normal physiology, 78, 85; in patient-physician relationship, 223

Empathy, 66, 255n4

Emperor's Medical Classic, 35

Endorphins, 100, 101, 251–252n4

Engel, George, 58, 234

Enlightenment, 184

Entralgo, Lain, 229, 235

Ernst, Edzard, 41

Ethics: clinical trials and, 17–18, 19–20, 247–248n3; Hippocratic oath and, 218–220; patient autonomy versus physician responsibility, 107–112, 119–120; truth-telling and, 113–124, 252n1

Ethnic medicine, 192–193. *See also* Culture

Expectations: and advertising OTC drugs, 40; and healing / pain relief, 102, 244; and patient-physician relationship, 47; placebos and, 16, 18, 73, 200, 201–202, 207, 208, 240

Fact, definition of, 24

Faith: healing, 165–168; religious, 69–70

Feyerabend, Paul, 194, 196

Fidelity, 217

Fitzgerald, F. S., 50

Flexner, Abraham, 187–188

Flexner Report, 7, 132, 187–188

Folklore, 157

Folk remedies, 144

Food, as medicine, 39

Food and Drug Administration (FDA), 17, 40, 148

Frank, Jerome, 137, 210

French Foreign Legion, 244

Fried, Charles, 224

Fixx, James, 253n5

Functional disease. *See* Illness

Galen, 161

Galton, Francis, 169

Gastroesophageal Reflux Disease (GERD), 231

Gate control theory, 97–98

Genetics, 52, 57

Glutamate, 98

Goddard, H. H., 132

Goethe, 189

Gordon, James, 145

Grand rounds, 67–68

Greece, 159; ancient, 182–184

Green movement, 144

Group support, 172. *See also* Community

Guide to Power and Healing (Harner), 172

H-2 blockers, 27, 39–40

Hahn, Robert, 155, 159

Hahnemann, Samuel, 178, 254n3

Harner, Michael, 172

Harrington, Ann, 250n4

Hart, F. D., 94

Hawkins, Ann, 252n3

Hawkins v. *McGee*, 118

Hawthorne effect, 16–17

Healer's Art (Cassell), 136–137

Healing: care and, 15, 66; charismatic, 34; definition of, 8, 136–138; faith, 165–168; and mind-body connection, 75–77, 250n4, 253n2; and non-Western cultures, 155; positive attitudes and, 104, 106–107; spontaneous regression, 74–75. *See also* Care; Placebos

Healing Heart (Cousins), 106

Health, defined, 51, 134–135

Health Insurance Plan of New York, 215

Heart disease and operations, 42–43, 85

Heisenberg, W., 202

Henderson, Lawrence, 108, 122

Herbal medicine, 139, 172

Hippocrates, 234

Hippocratic medicine, 160–161, 166, 182–183

Hippocratic oath, 218–219

Holism and Evolution (Smuts), 133

Holistic, defined, 133

Holistic Medical Association, 143

Library of Congress Cataloging-in-Publication Data

Spiro, Howard M. (Howard Marget), 1924–

    The power of hope : a doctor's perspective / Howard Spiro.

      p.   cm.

    "Prepared under the auspices of the Program for Humanities in Medicine, Yale University School of Medicine."

    "Portions of this book previously appeared in Doctors, patients, and placebos (Yale University Press, 1986)"—CIP t.p. verso.

    Includes bibliographical references and index.

    ISBN 0-300-07410-7 (alk. paper).—ISBN 0-300-07632-0 (pbk. : alk. paper)

    1. Medicine and psychology.   2. Hope—Psychological aspects.   3. Placebo (Medicine).   4. Sick—Psychology.   5. Mental healing.   6. Mind and body.   I. Title.

R726.5.S66   1998

610'.1'9—dc21   98-18731

                     CIP

The Power of Hope

A Doctor's Perspective

Howard Spiro, M.D.

In this book an eminent physician explores how patients and caring doctors can help lessen suffering when illness occurs. Dr. Howard Spiro urges that physicians focus on their patients' feelings of pain and anxiety as well as on physical symptoms. He also suggests that patients and their doctors be receptive to the emotional relief that may be obtained from nature and from hope.

Drawing on his previous highly praised work on the doctor-patient relationship and the problem of pain, Dr. Spiro tells how people can be helped by a combination of alternative medicine and mainstream medicine—a treatment of mind, body, and spirit that energizes patients, strengthens their expectations, and starts them on the road to feeling better. In various forms of alternative medicine, from meditation to massage, from faith healing to folk medicine, from herbology to homeopathy, practitioners heed patients' complaints and help them to help themselves.

Dr. Spiro encourages physicians to talk and listen to their patients as much as they look and measure, to treat the whole patient and not just the disease, and to integrate a scientific approach to medicine with alternative approaches that may alleviate pain and suffering.

"This book offers significant insights into the promise that alternative medicine offers to those who are ill. It is an important and timely contribution by one of the world's foremost gastroenterologists and clinicians."—Joseph Jacobs, M.D., former director, Office of Alternative Medicine, National Institutes of Health

Howard Spiro, M.D., professor of medicine at Yale University School of Medicine and director of the Program for Humanities in Medicine there, established the gastrointestinal section at Yale University School of Medicine in 1955. He is the author of *Clinical Gastroenterology*, now in its fourth edition, and *Doctors, Patients, and Placebos*. He is coeditor of *Empathy and the Practice of Medicine* and *Facing Death*, both published by Yale University Press, and *When Doctors Get Sick*.

Prepared under the auspices of the Program for Humanities in Medicine, Yale University School of Medicine